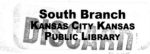

South Branch
KANSAS CITY KANSAS
PUBLIC LIBRARY
DISCARD

PRAISE FOR JOE FRIEL

"Joe Friel is arguably the most experienced perso

"Joe Friel is one of the world's foremost experts or

—*OUTSIDE* MAGAZINE

"Joe Friel's wealth of knowledge in triathlon is astounding and he has a wonderful way of sharing that knowledge with all athletes from beginners to elite professionals."

—SIRI LINDLEY, TRIATHLON WORLD CHAMPION

"Years of active multisport coaching have proven that Joe Friel has an unprecedented understanding of endurance sports. . . . Joe's professional approach and practical understanding of sports physiology has helped many endurance athletes of all abilities reach their full athletic potential."

—SIMON LESSING, FIVE-TIME TRIATHLON WORLD CHAMPION

"To say that Joe Friel knows a thing or two about how to ride a bicycle and stay fast would be a severe understatement."

—*ROAD BIKE ACTION*

PRAISE FOR *THE TRIATHLETE'S TRAINING BIBLE*

"What Tim Noakes's *Lore of Running* was for running, Friel's *Triathlete's Training Bible* is for triathlon."

—*RUNNER'S WORLD*

"*The Triathlete's Training Bible* is a fantastic guide. You can't go wrong using the advice in this book."

—SCOTT "THE TERMINATOR" MOLINA, PROFESSIONAL TRIATHLETE

"*The Triathlete's Training Bible* combines scientific research with the experience of a top endurance coach to provide the best training resource book available."

—GALE BERNHARDT, 2004 TEAM USA OLYMPIC TRIATHLON HEAD COACH

"Joe Friel has spent most of his life in devotion to the understanding and teaching of sport. Joe has managed to focus on the key components to athletic success while weeding out the noise. This book will play a substantial role in helping you take the next step as a triathlete." —JUSTIN DAERR, PROFESSIONAL TRIATHLETE

"As a triathlon coach, 2004 Olympian, and former top-ranked triathlete in the world, I've used *The Triathlete's Training Bible* as one of my key references. Joe Friel's training books have made the once 'crazy' sport of triathlon accessible to the public while also guiding seasoned athletes to their full potential."

—BARB LINDQUIST, 2004 OLYMPIC TRIATHLETE

"Whether you're a beginning triathlete or a seasoned pro, Joe Friel is the leading authority on triathlon training."

—RYAN BOLTON, IRONMAN WINNER, 2000 USA OLYMPIC TEAM, AND BOLTON ENDURANCE COACH

"*The Triathlete's Training Bible* can help you train for any distance and is most useful to newbies and self-trained athletes who want traditional training advice."

—*LIBRARY JOURNAL*

PRAISE FOR *THE CYCLIST'S TRAINING BIBLE*

"*The Cyclist's Training Bible* will have you systematically training just as world-class cyclists do. If you scrupulously follow its guidelines, I'm confident your racing performance will dramatically improve." —TUDOR BOMPA, PHD

"I find Friel's book a treasure of information for cyclists of all levels."

—ANDY HAMPSTEN, 1988 GIRO D'ITALIA WINNER,
1992 TOUR DE FRANCE STAGE WINNER AT ALPE D'HUEZ

"Nothing else comes close to *The Cyclist's Training Bible*'s comprehensive approach to planning out a season, creating a training schedule and incorporating diet and resistance training to an overall plan." —BIKERUMOR.COM

"Packed with worksheets, charts, visuals and a dense index and references for further reading, *The Cyclist's Training Bible* is an arsenal of encyclopedic information for ambitious riders." —DAILYPELOTON.COM

PRAISE FOR *FAST AFTER 50*

"*Fast After 50* is the best of this year's batch of practical books on science and performance. . . . Solid advice, clearly presented." *—RUNNER'S WORLD*

"*Fast After 50* is a gold mine of accessible info for all athletes and possibly the newest bible for the aging athlete." *—CANADIAN RUNNING*

"Read *Fast After 50* to learn more about the effects of aging on athletic performance and how you can be a competitive endurance athlete as you get older." *—TRIATHLETE* MAGAZINE

"*Fast After 50* continues to be a boon for the many cyclists looking to stay fit as they age." *—ROAD BIKE ACTION*

"*Fast After 50* might change your mindset and give you a new lease on life. . . . A smart approach to warding off the effects of age." *—ATHLETICS WEEKLY*

"Cyclists set on defying the aging process will want to get their hands on Joe Friel's *Fast After 50*." *—CANADIAN CYCLING* MAGAZINE

RIDE INSIDE

THE ESSENTIAL GUIDE TO GET THE MOST OUT OF INDOOR CYCLING, SMART TRAINERS, CLASSES, AND APPS

JOE FRIEL

WITH JIM RUTBERG

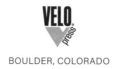

BOULDER, COLORADO

Copyright © 2020 by Joe Friel and Jim Rutberg

All rights reserved. Printed in the United States of America.

No part of this book may be reproduced, stored in a retrieval system, or
transmitted, in any form or by any means, electronic or photocopy or otherwise,
without the prior written permission of the publisher except in the case of brief
quotations within critical articles and reviews.

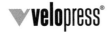

4745 Walnut Street, Unit A
Boulder, CO 80301-2587 USA

VeloPress is the leading publisher of books on endurance sports and is a division
of Pocket Outdoor Media. Focused on cycling, triathlon, running, swimming,
and nutrition/diet, VeloPress books help athletes achieve their goals of going
faster and farther. Preview books and contact us at velopress.com.

Distributed in the United States and Canada by Ingram Publisher Services

A Cataloging-in-Publication record for this book is available from the
Library of Congress. ISBN 978-1-948007-13-9

This paper meets the requirements of ANSI/NISO Z39.48-1992
(Permanence of Paper).

Art direction by Vicki Hopewell
Cover photo courtesy of Wahoo Fitness
Cover and interior design by Lisa Williams

20 21 22 / 10 9 8 7 6 5 4 3 2 1

CONTENTS

FOREWORD
BY STEPHEN SEILER, PHD

My indoor cycling adventure began three years ago in a hospital waiting room. I sat there with a swollen, painful leg waiting to start blood tests and diagnostic imagery. The testing revealed a large blood clot in my thigh, which explained why walking to the mailbox made my blood- and oxygen-starved lower leg feel like I was running repeat 400m sprints. The blood tests also revealed that I had a genetic disorder that made me very vulnerable, when I acted like my years of training had made me impregnable. Years of sitting in meetings at a university, not having time to exercise the way I was used to, and lots of birthdays under my belt had conspired against me. So, as I waited for the nurse, I opened Google and plotted a revolution. The furniture of an upstairs TV room would be thrown out and training equipment would be brought in. Daily doses of efficient exercise were needed, and I began searching for the right training tools.

Today, I have a small home training room equipped with kettlebells, a barbell wedged into a corner with weights on one end, elastic bands, weight vests, a ski-poling ergometer, and a bicycle trainer. I use them all to varying degrees, but my bicycle trainer is the most important investment I have made. It's the most-used training device I own and by far the most fun! I designed my home gym to be efficient. What I did not expect was how exciting and enjoyable training and sweating all alone in that room would become. Turns out that I am not alone at all. No matter what day of the week or time of day I ride, I am always connected to cyclists all over the world!

Since you are reading this, you must be planning on joining me and millions of other indoor cycling enthusiasts. Like everything else, there is a learning curve when it comes to indoor cycling. Those old rickety bicycle trainers you may have imagined are a thing of the past. Modern indoor trainers are high tech and well engineered. They are also more complicated than those old spin bikes! What are the right settings? What the heck is a "PowerUp"? Where does my ride data go? What is "erg-mode"? Is a one-hour ride inside the same as a one-hour ride outside? Why am I sweating so much?

In the last 18 months, I have logged over 500 hours on my indoor trainer. It took me quite a long time to figure out the rules and the tools of riding inside, making the connections easier, the training more effective, and the group rides and races even more motivating and fun. Thanks to Joe Friel and *Ride Inside*, your learning curve will be much faster than mine.

Pardon the pun, but Joe Friel knows endurance training inside and out. He has been teaching smart endurance training for decades through his books and coaching services. Now he has written the go-to companion for anyone who is new to riding inside. Whether you're young or old, out of shape or age-group champion, he will guide you through all the technology choices and issues, the differences between cycling indoors and outdoors, and how to design a training plan that works within your time and life constraints.

I am a sports scientist, so I try to understand how the body works. Despite 30 years of active research and a competitive background in numerous sports, I have never felt more in tune with my own body and how it responds to training than I do now because of the effectiveness and control I have when I train indoors. Turn the pages of *Ride Inside* and I am confident that you will not only unlock a fantastic tool for fitness, but also open a window into your own body and how it works. Good luck!

INTRODUCTION

I never thought I would choose to ride inside on a sunny spring morning, but there I was, swinging my leg over the top tube to ride for an hour in front of a computer monitor. I still love to ride outside, and that's where you'll find nearly all the cycling events and triathlons we train for, but recent improvements in the technology, community, and convenience of indoor cycling have made riding inside more appealing than ever. I had a great indoor ride on that day, and many since, to the point that riding inside is a regular component of my training, regardless of the weather outside.

I'm certainly not the only one who feels more drawn to riding inside than I used to be. Truth be told, I'm not what you would call an "early adopter" in the indoor cycling scene. I've been a cyclist and triathlete for decades, and now that I'm in my 70s I have more free time to schedule my day around the best time to ride outside. As a coach, however, it is clear to me that over the past 10 years, technological advances in indoor cycling have elevated a frankly second-rate training alternative to an essential tool that can offer significant advantages over training outdoors. These days, riding inside isn't what you do when the weather is too miserable to ride outside; it's what you do when you want a great workout.

Although indoor trainers and studio-based cycling classes have been around for decades, the new indoor cycling revolution started with the development of electronic "smart" trainers. The clunky "dumb" trainers of the past were replaced by devices that could monitor and control the resistance the rider feels. Apps like Zwift, TrainerRoad, The Sufferfest, Rouvy, and FulGaz then threw gas on the fire by streaming training content, connecting riders across town and around the world, and allowing cyclists to ride together in virtual worlds. For many athletes, the days of grinding out a ride alone on a noisy "dumb" trainer are just a distant memory.

Given how competitive cyclists and triathletes are, it didn't take long for riders to start organizing their own virtual races on Zwift and similar apps. By 2018, local clubs were hosting online race series, and pro teams started realizing that virtual group rides and e-races were an opportunity for fans to interact with their favorite pros and for the team to provide value to sponsors. Today, well over half a million riders from all over the globe have raced virtually since virtual racing was introduced. Riding inside, you can test your fitness against a group of your athletic peers—from anywhere in the world—any time of day or night, all without the worries of flatting, crashing, or getting run over.

Interest in indoor cycling and e-racing surged in early 2020 when a global pandemic forced people around the world to stay at home to slow the spread of a highly contagious virus. Everything outside, from local group rides to professional bike races, was cancelled. In some areas of Europe, even recreational cycling was prohibited. During March and April 2020, a time of year when file uploads from virtual training platforms normally declines, the online coaching service provider TrainingPeaks experienced a 500 percent increase in the number of Zwift file uploads compared to the same period in 2019.

Virtual racing seems likely to have an ongoing presence in the future of professional cycling. Grand tour organizers have considered running their prologues on smart trainers, as have organizers of some spring classics road races. Pros raced each other in the Zwift Tour for All "stage race" during the COVID-19 pandemic. There's even been talk of establishing e-racing as an Olympic sport. In professional cycling, races are struggling largely because they must compete with other sports for sponsorship. And the costs of putting on a pro race are exorbitant and continue to increase. Compared with coordinating road closures, police assistance, barricades, portable toilet rentals, and everything that goes into putting on a live event, the production costs for e-races are quite low. Granted, it's not quite the same as having fans along the road cheering on their favorite riders, but that isn't stopping those who see a future for online racing.

In the not-too-distant future, I foresee a computer app that will put you virtually on the start line during a livestream of the real outdoor Tour de France—or any other race. You may not be able to literally compete as part of the Tour de France peloton, but you could see how you stack up against some of the best riders in the world in the most famous bike races on the planet. Even if you don't last long, virtually rolling with the pros would be an experience fans of stick-and-ball sports could never replicate.

Well, enough daydreaming about racing the Tour de France from your living room. You don't have to race to reap the benefits of riding inside. When it comes to fitness, riding indoor smart trainers actually works better than being on the road for some rides. You can do preprogrammed workouts uploaded to your trainer without traffic, stoplights, or dogs chasing you. Want to ride flat terrain or a series of mountain climbs? Go ahead. Just select your course. Short days and icy roads in the winter? No problem. Limited time for a ride? You can wedge in a quick workout between other activities without having a long haul to a suitable course. And if you're training while recovering from injury, you can ride inside without the risk of crashing again. Some apps now even allow you to talk with your coach or other riders during the workout. Riding inside has become so convenient and appealing that some athletes have become inside-only cyclists who only ride outdoors on special occasions.

There's never been a better time to start riding inside or to use indoor cycling to augment your outdoor training. And there's so much more coming in terms of technology, connectivity, community, and competition. But I won't get into more pie-in-the-sky daydreams in this book. Instead, I'll lead you through what you need to know to get the most out of riding inside—and to enjoy it. Along the way, I hope to answer many of your questions about indoor cycling, including:

- How do you blend indoor and outdoor fitness?
- Are there any physiological differences between riding inside and outside?
- What equipment and technology do you need to get started riding inside?
- How should you set up your indoor training space?

- How do you make your inside training purposefully mesh with your outside races or other events?
- Should your training be planned any differently for inside versus outside riding?
- How do you get started in virtual group rides or e-racing?
- What workouts can you do indoors to make the best use of your training time?

So, are you ready to ride inside? Let's get started.

WHY RIDE A BIKE INDOORS?

More athletes than ever are joining the indoor cycling movement. Experienced outdoor cyclists are moving indoors, new cyclists are gaining the fitness and confidence to participate in outdoor events and group rides, and busy cyclists who had given up on the idea of being fit and powerful are discovering the pathway back to the athletes they want to be. This book is for all of you, including indoor cyclists who want to perform at your best and have no intention or desire to ride outside.

There was a time, not long ago, when I would do just about anything to avoid riding inside. My strong aversion stemmed from decades in the Dark Ages of Indoor Cycling, winters spent staring at the wall or Tour de France replays in a damp basement or freezing garage. The equipment seemed equally medieval—either a rack of cold rollers strapped together with a rubber hose, or a contraption somewhere between a vice and thumbscrew mercilessly squeezing the rear axle. Indoor cycling was a last resort, not a first choice.

Plenty has changed since then, and we have now entered the Golden Era of Indoor Cycling. The whole ecosystem for riding inside has shifted. Where there was once isolation, there is now a worldwide community. Where there was once boredom, there is now engagement and excitement. And perhaps most important for performance-oriented cyclists, ambiguity about the physical work being performed has been replaced by data-driven certainty.

In early 2020, the appeal of indoor cycling also got a massive boost from a most unfortunate set of circumstances. As a novel coronavirus (COVID-19) swept across the world, societies everywhere realized isolation and "flattening the curve" were the best ways to slow the virus's transmission and prevent health-care systems from being overwhelmed. Entire countries enacted "stay at home" orders that shut down all but essential businesses, closed schools and universities, and restricted nonessential travel. In Italy and Spain, outdoor cycling for anything more than transportation was prohibited for a time. In the United States, group rides and all endurance sports events were prohibited.

People in the US were encouraged to get outside for walks, hikes, runs, and bike rides, and many people dusted off old bikes in their garages and rode for the first time in years. Some bike shops experienced an increase in business, and companies selling indoor trainers and indoor cycling apps saw tremendous growth. A lot of cyclists and triathletes turned to Zwift, The Sufferfest, Trainer-Road, Road Grand Tours (RGT Cycling), Rouvy, Bkool, and other indoor cycling apps to continue training with power, take advantage of the benefits of smart trainers, and stay engaged with other athletes in their communities.

In the chapters to come, I will show you how to integrate proven sports science, the latest indoor cycling equipment, cutting-edge technologies, and your athletic goals and identity to help you become a faster and stronger cyclist. My aim is not to take you off the road, track, or trail, but rather to improve your performance everywhere you ride. Likewise, it is important to recognize indoor cycling as its own discipline and not always an alternative or prelude to riding outside.

A good portion of this book will teach you how to plan a period or season of indoor cycling to meet your athletic goals. To effectively improve your cycling performance or overall fitness, you need a plan that moves you to new performance peaks. A well-designed training plan and library of workouts are tools to help you get there.

WHY RIDE INSIDE?

There are so many good reasons to ride inside today. In fact, the wide variety of athletes doing indoor cycling bring an equally diverse set of reasons to participate. People new to cycling are discovering interactive bikes and programs like Peloton® or rigorous indoor group classes such as SoulCycle. Amateur cyclists and triathletes are incorporating structured indoor workouts into their annual training plans—not just when the weather is uncooperative. Elite and professional athletes are relying on the predictability, control, and safety of indoor cycling to prepare for events worldwide. An increasing number of athletes are competing indoors in e-racing, using smart trainers and internet-connected apps to race virtually against real competitors from all over this world in whole new worlds created by software engineers. All of these riders have their own motivations or circumstances that led them indoors. In many cases, riding inside isn't just an alternative to riding outside, but a better choice.

TIME MANAGEMENT

If it seems like the world is moving faster and there are more demands on your time than ever before, welcome to being an adult in the 21st century. Time is a limiting factor for almost every amateur cyclist or triathlete I work with. Unless you are making a living as a professional athlete, you have to make time for your career and sport.

In addition to work and sport, there are relationships you need to stay engaged with. Your spouse or partner, your kids, and your friends are important for your long-term health and happiness, and they are also integral parts of your athletic support system. Just as training stress needs to be balanced with adequate rest, the time and dedication you commit to training needs to be balanced with attention to the relationships that help make that training time available.

Room for Your Priorities

With all the competing priorities in our lives, time is a precious resource. Training indoors can be advantageous because it is so time-efficient. You don't have to spend time doing the mental gymnastics of figuring out which layers you need to wear for the weather. You don't have to hunt for your one missing arm warmer (there's always one . . .). There's no reason to think about choosing a ride route that will fit with the goals of your workout. Depending on your indoor setup, the equipment can be left ready to go day after day. All you need to do is step into a chamois, slip on your cycling shoes, and clip in.

A Focus on Workout Execution

Competitive cyclists and triathletes race outdoors (although e-sports are creating opportunities to compete indoors), and the workouts required to build fitness require focus. When training outdoors, can you give everything you have for a high-intensity interval, or do you have to hold something back and reserve some focus for watching out for cars, kids, dogs, curves, and stop signs? Indoors, you are guaranteed to have the control to execute long intervals uninterrupted. You can stay in an aerodynamic position for long period of time, which is key for adapting to the position so you can be both aero and powerful. And you can ride yourself cross-eyed and heaving, if you want to, without losing your balance and drifting into traffic or off the road. Generally speaking, the more focus your workout requires, the better it is to do indoors. You can build the engine indoors, and then go outdoors and develop the skills to use it.

Proximity to Terrain

Perhaps the biggest time saver is the fact that you don't have to ride to a location where you can start your workout. For many urban and suburban athletes, that can take 30 minutes or more of riding roads and paths dotted with stop signs, traffic lights, congested traffic, hostile drivers, and road infrastructure which was not designed with bicycles in mind.

If you have an interval set that lasts 40 minutes, but it takes 30 minutes each way to get to a road, bike path, or trail safe enough to execute it, your ride has to be a minimum of 100 minutes. Add in the time to get dressed and get the gear ready, plus the time at the end to reverse the process, and you have to budget at least 2 hours to accomplish a 40-minute interval set. Of course, that's not all time wasted, as there is certainly a benefit to those 60 minutes of riding to and from the location for your interval set. But when you only have 60–90 minutes available that day, you need an alternative. When you ride indoors, you are on course immediately, ready for the interval after just a quick warm-up.

Convenience for Workday Training

As much as I love lunch rides, they can be a logistical headache. In comparison, going out for a run in the middle of a workday is pretty easy: You need a bag with your running shoes and a change of clothes, and a towel for your shower. To go on a lunch ride, you have to get the bike to the office, along with your helmet and shoes and associated gear, and you have to have a secure place to keep the bike. If you're lucky, you work in an organization that supports bike commuting and has secure, indoor bike storage and shower facilities (whether you ride in or bring the bike on your car). Unfortunately, many workplaces are not so bike friendly.

An increasing number of workplaces have indoor workout facilities on-site or a cycling studio nearby. By eliminating the hassle and time to schlep a bike and bulky gear to and from the office (assuming you're not commuting by bike already), indoor cycling makes a lunch ride as gear-intensive as a midday run.

READY 24 HOURS A DAY

Riding inside liberates cyclists from being confined to the hours between sunrise and sunset. The freedom to get on the trainer at any time of day or night is the only thing that makes endurance training possible for some people. Oftentimes, the early morning is the only part of the day that an athlete can really control. Once the day gets started, other priorities may take precedence, like taking kids to school, getting to work on time, and shuffling around to meetings, pickups, and appointments. And that's when the day goes as planned, which is . . . never. More likely, there's a project that needs to be finished, a deadline that must be met, a kid with a fever who needs to be taken out of school, or even an opportunity to catch up with an old friend you haven't seen for a long time.

The early morning, before dawn and before everyone else gets up and gets in the way, is your time. This has been the secret to success for thousands of high-performance cyclists, runners, and triathletes who also happen to be executives and working parents.

Maybe mornings aren't your thing or they just don't fit into your schedule. The indoor trainer will be there in the evenings too. There are even training strategies that may make evening workouts particularly beneficial by taking advantage of certain aspects of nutrition. For instance, training when you have low carbohydrate availability is a strategy some athletes use to improve fat oxidation. But to do it, you have to deplete muscle glycogen stores. One way to accomplish that is to do a hard ride with high-carbohydrate availability in the evening, consume adequate total calories but little carbohydrate before bed, and then complete an endurance or moderate-intensity ride in the morning. You'll start the morning workout without replenishing muscle glycogen stores, which means training with low carbohydrate availability.

CHILDCARE

One of the hardest times to be an athlete is when your children are too young to be left alone. Depending on the kid(s), that can be well into the teenage years. In many two-parent households, one parent can sneak out for a ride while the other is at home. But as life gets busier, both parents have things to do, and the tag-team strategy breaks down. For single-parent households, the challenge can be exponentially greater. In both scenarios, hiring babysitters is an option, albeit an expensive one. Pulling small children in a trailer is an option too, but it comes with a whole raft of additional considerations.

Indoor cycling can be a training savior for parents. With babies and toddlers in the house, naptime can be an opportunity to jump on the trainer (if you're not taking a nap yourself, or doing any of the other thousand things on your list). Early mornings can be a good option when you have school-aged kids in the house. Regardless of where you squeeze in the time, riding inside while your kids are home has the secondary benefit of modeling healthy exercise habits and showing your children that exercise can be a lifelong activity. You could even make the argument that riding inside works better for this purpose because children actually observe you performing the activity, rather than just seeing you leave for extended periods of time and come back sweaty.

SOCIAL ENGAGEMENT

In the Dark Ages of Indoor Cycling, we were confined to basements, garages, and laundry rooms, with no way to connect to our friends and training partners who were doing the same thing in their basements, garages, and laundry rooms. Training with a partner or in a group increases accountability, which reduces the likelihood that you'll skip a ride. Many athletes also find they can push themselves harder or complete more total work if they are with someone else. Group rides, indoor cycling classes, and rides with a couple of friends are also large components of an athlete's social group. Now, with smart trainers and stationary bikes connected to interactive training platforms, you can reap the social and performance benefits of group training without leaving the basement.

ENVIRONMENTAL FACTORS

Fresh air and sunlight on your face are two of life's greatest joys, but sometimes the air isn't so fresh and the sunlight is too harsh. It is sad to have to say this, but in some environmental conditions, riding inside is better for your health.

Air Quality

Particulate pollution (chemicals released from many human activities) is a problem for any creature with lungs, and the amount of air you're pulling into your lungs per hour has an impact on the amount of pollution you're inhaling. Compared to a sedentary population that spends less than an hour a day outdoors breathing unfiltered air, endurance athletes spend hundreds more hours each year outdoors breathing at least 10 times the volume of air. Perhaps worse than the duration and volume, you breathe far deeper during exercise, exposing more lung tissue to pollutants.

As a matter of perspective, the positive cardiovascular health benefits of aerobic exercise far outweigh any potential risk of lung disease from rapid breathing during exercise. However, when air quality is particularly bad and levels of particulate pollution are high, athletes need to recognize that strenuous exercise exposes them to exponentially more pollution. Athletes with lung disease or asthma will be even more affected as air quality deteriorates. The lesson here is to take smog alerts and air thick with forest fire smoke seriously, and ride inside when air quality is poor. For athletes living in densely populated urban areas, this can represent a significant number of days per year.

Sun Exposure

Some sun exposure is important for athletes—and everyone, in fact—because sunlight helps our bodies manufacture vitamin D, and it's much easier to make the vitamin D you need than it is to consume it through food. On the other hand, a lifetime of long days outside under the blazing sun can lead to skin damage and increase the risk of developing skin cancer. Many of us who have been endurance athletes for many decades started training well before the long-term risks of sun exposure were well-known, and we have already accumulated quite a lot of damage. Some athletes with sensitive skin, athletes who already have skin conditions related to sun exposure, and athletes taking medications (including some antibiotics, antihistamines, and even NSAID painkillers) that can cause sun sensitivity for some people, may benefit from spending more time riding indoors.

SAFETY

More than any of the factors above, safety is the biggest reason a growing number of cyclists prefer to ride inside. The number of automobile-crash fatalities has been declining for 40 years, but the number of pedestrian and cyclist deaths from traffic collisions has been increasing in recent years. According to a 2019 report from the National Transportation Safety Board (NTSB), 857 cyclists were killed in 2018, the most since 1990. From 2017 to 2018, there was a 6.3 percent increase in the number of cyclists killed, despite a decrease of 2.4 percent in the total number of traffic deaths in the US during the same period.

Depending on where you live, these trends bring either good news or bad news. Urban cycling, on the one hand, is getting more dangerous. According to the same report, from 2009 to 2018 there has been a 48 percent increase in cyclist fatalities in urban areas. But rural areas have seen a decrease of 8.9 percent. This trend holds true for pedestrians and all vehicle types, although urban pedestrians and cyclists were most affected. As many US cities have grown and become more auto-centric, getting around in them has become more dangerous.

Distracted driving is epidemic, with drivers looking down at their phones and navigating dashboard touch screens, but it's not the only reason cyclists are dying outdoors. As cars and trucks get bigger, particularly in terms of the height of the hood, collisions with "non-occupants" get more deadly. Instead of potentially rolling up onto the hood, you're more likely to be run over. The combination of an increased number of urban cyclists and an increase in truck and delivery vehicle traffic is proving deadly in big cities. In New York City, 29 cyclists were killed in traffic collisions in 2019 (more than double the number in 2018), and 25 of them were killed by drivers of large trucks, buses, SUVs, or vans.

Overall, I remain hopeful about the safety of outdoor cycling. I understand why cyclists are afraid, especially because media and social media make us more aware of collisions and fatalities around the country and the world. Statistics don't mean a whole lot when it's someone you know who gets hit, and the statistics don't include all the close calls, harassing maneuvers, and hostile drivers that cyclists encounter on a regular basis. Nonetheless, I believe e-bikes and other micromobility technologies (electric scooters, etc.), along with increased congestion and reduced parking, will encourage more people to ride bicycles and get out of cars, and that there will be more pressure on communities to create and upgrade infrastructure to make "non-occupants" safer. For performance cyclists who ride out into more rural areas, I'm hopeful that automotive technology eventually overcomes our human flaws of inattention and distractibility.

BENEFITS TO YOUR HEALTH, FITNESS, AND COMPETITIVE EDGE

When you really stop and think about it, there are lot of advantages to riding inside, but most of them fall into the category of "avoiding a negative." Indoors, you won't get hit by a car, get lost, get home late, get caught in a thunderstorm, run out of daylight, run out of water, or mess up an interval workout because you reached the top of the hill too soon. But riding inside isn't about what won't happen; it's about what can happen.

YOU GET FASTER

There is perhaps no greater proof that riding inside can prepare you for winning performances outdoors than Mathew Hayman's victory at the 2016 Paris–Roubaix. For those less familiar with European cycling, Paris–Roubaix is one of professional cycling's five Monuments, prestigious one-day races that are very long (150–165 miles) and exquisitely brutal. Paris–Roubaix's vicious reputation stems from more than two dozen stretches of rough Napoleonic-era cobblestone roads, which gradually rattle, bounce, and batter riders into submission, with crash wounds to prove it.

To even be in contention to win Paris–Roubaix, a rider first needs to be strong enough and lucky enough to last through the battle of attrition and reach the final 40 miles with the front group. Your ability to succeed from there forward, however, depends a lot on how much the preceding hours took out of you. When you're more fit, you don't have to dig as deep into your reserves as often or as much as the other riders, so you have something left to give when it matters most.

Australian Mathew Hayman was a journeyman professional cyclist. He was strong and smart, and he was one of the best teammates a leader could have. He didn't win many races and wasn't the most famous rider, but his work as a teammate put a lot of champions atop podiums around the world. Going into 2016, he had ridden Paris–Roubaix 15 times and finished them all. It was his favorite race, and because it's such a battle of attrition, it is one of the races where journeyman team players can ride themselves into the leadership role if they're the rider who makes it into the front group.

In a race called Omloop Het Nieuwsblad in late February, Hayman broke his arm in a crash. He had been training for months with the plan to be in top shape for Paris–Roubaix on April 11, but with a broken arm, he couldn't train outdoors and certainly couldn't compete in other spring races that are both goal events and major training stimuli. In his 17th year as a professional cyclist, it looked like his spring classics season was finished before it started.

Determined not to lose the fitness he had worked so hard to gain, Hayman rode more than 1,000 kilometers (624 miles) on an indoor trainer in his garage while his broken arm healed. Just like he would have outdoors, he rode a lot of hours at a moderate pace and completed focused interval workouts prescribed by his coach to keep and develop the power required to ride Paris–Roubaix.

On the day of the race, Hayman wasn't designated as the leader, the rider the team was going to work for and hopefully put in a position to win. That was normal, as was his role as "road captain," the rider charged with adjusting the team's tactics on the fly. As the race unfolded, his experience and tactical prowess helped him make all the right decisions about when to go hard, when to chase, and whom to follow, and he made it into the final 20 miles as the last team rider in the lead group.

After nearly six hours of racing, Hayman and Tom Boonen, already a four-time winner of Paris–Roubaix, rode onto the velodrome in Roubaix with a lap and a half to go and a chase group of three close behind. In the final 500 meters, the group of five were all together, and Hayman was at the front, with his face in the wind rather than in the slipstream behind. Starting the sprint from the front with Tom Boonen, Edvald Boasson Hagen, Sep Vanmarcke, and Ian Stannard in your draft would normally be the worst possible choice, but this time it worked, and Hayman had enough left in the tank to capture the biggest win of his career.

Though Hayman's path to Paris–Roubaix victory was an anomaly, there is an argument to be made that the advantages of indoor cycling I mentioned earlier actually enhanced his preparation. Compared to other riders who were traveling and training and getting battered in other brutal races, Hayman was at home training when and how he wanted to, eating the food he chose, sleeping in his own bed, and spending time with his family. Precise training, great recovery, and a low-stress environment. Beat that.

YOU GET HEALTHIER

If you are an experienced cycling or triathlon competitor, you are already experiencing the health benefits associated with improved cardiorespiratory fitness. For those who are newer to endurance training, and as a review for everyone, it is important to understand the relationship between exercise and health.

I have spent my career helping endurance athletes improve performance, which is not necessarily synonymous with improving health. At the elite end of the spectrum, athletes are pushing themselves to the point where their immune systems can be compromised and where they risk various musculoskeletal injuries. Certainly, one of my goals as a coach is to help them optimize performance without those negative outcomes, but in principle it's important to recognize that athletes focused primarily on competitive performance may willingly accept some increased health risks.

For most amateur athletes, the net benefits of exercise for improving long-term health far outweigh the risks associated with being sedentary. Here are just a few of the health benefits of exercise.

Reduced Risk of Cardiovascular Disease

Exercise—both aerobic exercise and resistance training—is unquestionably effective for reducing the risk of cardiovascular disease. Compared to sedentary populations, people who exercise regularly (at least 150 minutes a week) have substantially lower risks for developing high blood pressure or suffering a stroke or heart attack.

For some athletes, though, too much of a good thing may be harmful. As a large generation reaches the 50+ age group, more people are experiencing cardiac arrythmia, particularly various types of tachycardia characterized by rapid heart rates. Decades of high-intensity exercise may be a contributing factor for developing tachycardia, particularly atrial fibrillation, in some athletes.

Stronger Immune System

Exercise causes inflammation and also raises your body's anti-inflammatory response. Acute (temporary) inflammation caused by exercise is a necessary part of the process that leads to greater fitness. It is also the immune system's healthy response to allergens and infections. With a healthy immune system, your body's anti-inflammatory mechanisms restore homeostasis once the threat has passed. On the other hand, chronic inflammation is thought to play a role in the development of cardiovascular disease, type 2 diabetes, arthritis, and even dementia. But people who exercise regularly and have greater aerobic fitness are less likely to experience chronic inflammation.

During the COVID-19 public health crisis, the interaction between training and immunity became a hot topic for coaches and athletes. It is well established that exercise supports a healthy and functional immune system better than being sedentary, but athletes wondered whether high-volume or high-intensity exercise potentially suppressed immune function and increased susceptibility to infection. The short answer is that individual bouts of exercise are unlikely to increase infection risk, but dramatic and sustained increases in training workload can be a contributing factor, along with disturbed or insufficient sleep, insufficient energy intake, elevated lifestyle stress, and more (see Chapter 9).

Reduced Risk of Type 2 Diabetes

According to the most recent National Diabetes Statistics Report from the Centers for Disease Control and Prevention (CDC), more than 34.2 million Americans (10.5 percent of the population) had diabetes in 2018. Of them, about 90–95 percent had type 2 diabetes, where the pancreas produces insufficient insulin to adequately control blood sugar levels. The causes of type 2 diabetes are largely associated with lifestyle, in contrast to type 1 diabetes, which is an autoimmune reaction that destroys some or all of the insulin-producing cells in the pancreas. Exercise reduces the risk of developing type 2 diabetes by increasing insulin sensitivity and increasing your capacity to store ingested carbohydrates as muscle glycogen.

Improved Cognitive Function

You can view this benefit as "exercise makes you smarter" or "exercise prevents cognitive decline." Both are likely true. Exercise improves circulation and oxygen delivery to the brain, which promotes neurogenesis. It also improves neuroplasticity, or the ability to learn and retain new skills. Two types of exercise are important for cognitive function: Aerobic exercise improves global cognition and executive functioning via cardiovascular benefits. Exercises that challenge your motor skills (complex tasks, balance, coordination) and require keeping track of information (interval training) are also important because they directly improve task-specific neuroplasticity. In another case of "use it or lose it," exercise has also been shown to protect against cognitive decline associated with aging.

YOU LOSE WEIGHT

In endurance sports that involve hills and mountains, body weight plays a significant role in performance. Being lighter means you don't have as much mass to move against gravity. That doesn't mean being as lean as possible is automatically the best option for endurance athletes. When athletes become too lean, physical capacity to perform work can start to decrease, and athletes become more susceptible to illness and injury. If you are looking to lose weight, the goal is to reach a sustainable body weight that doesn't compromise your power output or immune system.

There are far more amateur athletes who have weight they can lose than there are athletes who are at risk of becoming dangerously lean. Indoor cycling can contribute to the energy expenditure side of the "calories in versus calories out" equation, particularly because you can expend upward of 1,000 calories during 60 minutes of high-intensity indoor cycling, whereas you're more likely to expend 500–600 calories at a less intense, endurance pace outdoors.

Truth be told, however, nutrition plays a more significant role than exercise when it comes to weight loss. It takes an hour of strenuous exercise to expend 1,000 calories, but you can consume a 2,000-calorie meal in 10 minutes. The old adage "you can't outrun a bad diet" is true. Where indoor cycling creates an advantage is the increased opportunity to exercise consistently.

YOU IMPROVE ENDURANCE PERFORMANCE EVERYWHERE

Just as Mathew Hayman used indoor cycling to maintain and improve his fitness for bike racing, athletes in other endurance sports can use indoor cycling to supplement their sport-specific training. This strategy can offer a way to increase an athlete's aerobic workload with less muscle damage (as cycling is low-impact and not weight-bearing). Similarly, it can be used to maintain aerobic fitness while a non-cyclist is recovering from a sport-specific injury, depending on the injury. Sport-specific training is essential for meeting the demands of your competition, but generalized aerobic training stress improves cardiorespiratory fitness that can be applied to any endurance activity.

YOU ADAPT TO HEAT

Heat acclimatization is essential for athletes training to compete in a hot or humid environment. When you live in Boulder, Colorado, through the winter and need to be ready for an early season goal race in Arizona or Southern California, it is a good idea to take proactive steps to adapt to exercising in the heat before you go. Triathletes often use heat acclimation strategies to prepare for the intense heat during the Ironman® World Championship in Kona, Hawaii, and ultrarunners use it to get ready for events like Western States and the Badwater 135, which goes through Death Valley in July.

There are specific heat acclimation protocols, typically incorporating both passive exposure to heat and training in a heated environment. Indoor cycling is one of the more convenient ways for athletes to exercise in a climate-controlled room. The outcomes athletes are looking for include lower resting core temperature, increased plasma volume, more rapid onset of sweating, increased sweat rate, decreased electrolyte concentration in sweat, and reduced sensations of thermal strain.

THE PROMISE OF RIDING INSIDE

There's no doubt that indoor cycling is an effective way to create, maintain, and improve cardiorespiratory fitness, cycling-specific power output, and long-term markers for physical and mental health. And there is no question that riding inside is more convenient, more time efficient, and safer than riding outside.

The only remaining question is: How do you get the most out of riding inside? In the coming chapters I will show you the science behind and the steps to building high-performance fitness, starting with the essential issue of how indoor and outdoor riding compare. You will learn how to structure workouts, training intensities, and training plans that specifically leverage the advantages of indoor cycling. In Chapter 5, you can explore the four different ways you can ride inside and the pros and cons of each. And finally, we'll bring it all together with guidance for getting the most out of the fitness gains from indoor cycling, whether you're competing inside or outside.

I've spent most of my life engaged in endurance training and coaching. I have witnessed a handful of game-changing training innovations in that time, and I am grateful I had the opportunity to play a role in some of them, such as sports drinks and sports nutrition products, heart rate monitors, power meters, training analysis software, and the professionalization of endurance coaching. Riding inside has been an integral part of cycling for more than a century, but only recently have the tools and technology existed to make indoor cycling so much more than a rainy day alternative to training outdoors. Riding inside is quickly becoming a substantial component of competitive cyclists' annual training plans, bringing busy cyclists back to the sport, inspiring new cyclists to start pedaling, and becoming a competitive discipline of its own. In the long run, I believe the developments we are living through now will be viewed as another game-changing step forward in endurance training and competition. So, let's get started and show you how to take advantage of this new landscape to improve your fitness and get an edge on your competition.

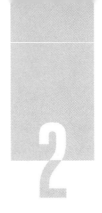

INDOORS AND OUTDOORS: WHAT'S DIFFERENT

Does it really make any difference if you ride inside or on the road or a trail? Does anything change in regard to how you interact with the bike? How about your fitness? Can you develop fitness in the same ways whether inside or out? There are in fact many advantages—and some disadvantages—to riding indoors thanks to how it differs from outdoor cycling. We'll start with physiology to understand what's happening in your body when you ride a bike inside or outside. Then we'll take a look at the mechanical interaction of the rider and the bike. Let's get started with the most basic matter—your fitness.

INDOOR FITNESS FOR OUTDOOR PERFORMANCE

Whether you are riding an indoor cycle, a bicycle on an indoor trainer, or a bicycle on the road, there are only three physiological determinants of fitness: *aerobic capacity*, *anaerobic threshold*, and *economy*. Every workout you do—from the very hardest to the very easiest—is intended to improve one or more of these markers of fitness (or at least it should be). By understanding what these are all about, you can make your workouts more focused on results and also come to appreciate the differences between riding indoors and outdoors. We'll come back to those differences after we first establish what fitness is.

AEROBIC CAPACITY

Just as with a car's engine, your body combines oxygen and fuel—mostly fat and carbohydrate—to make it possible for you to turn the cranks. And also like your car, the more oxygen you process, the faster you go. This concept is called aerobic capacity, or VO_2max. That's a shorthand term used by sport scientists to describe what aerobic capacity is all about—the *maximum volume of oxygen* you are capable of processing to produce energy. That energy, of course, is what allows you to turn the pedals on your bike.

There's one caveat here, however, that you need to be aware of: weight. This becomes apparent when you consider the units of measure in the scientific formula for VO_2max:

$$VO_2max = mL\ O_2\ /\ kg\ /\ min$$

Translated into everyday language, this means aerobic capacity is a consequence of how many milliliters (30 mL is about 1 fluid ounce) of oxygen you can process for your weight in kilograms. This is an indicator of your energy production capacity per minute when at your highest extended power output. "Weight" in this case means your body weight. But when riding outside, where gravity is a factor, weight includes your bike, shoes, helmet, clothing, water bottle, and anything else you're carrying along on the ride besides your body. But the technician testing you for VO_2max in the lab seldom considers all of the miscellaneous equipment and focuses only on your body weight.

Because the formula calls for dividing oxygen consumption by weight, the greater your weight, the lower your VO_2max. There's no doubt that you're very aware of this when climbing a hill: if you're carrying more weight up the hill, you'll go slower.

Among elite male cyclists, the typical VO_2max is in the high 70s to low 80s of milliliters of oxygen per kilogram per minute (OK, I'll stop using that formula from now on). Elite female athletes are typically about 10 percent lower. That's because they typically have a bit more body fat than men, percentagewise, which essentially increases their relative weight. VO_2max declines if we stop training. It also tends to drop with aging.

In a nutshell, that's aerobic capacity. So, how do you improve it with training? One way I'm sure you've already thought of is by decreasing weight—of both your body and your equipment. That's not always a good idea, though. If you're already pretty lean, then trying to get rid of a few more pounds can be counterproductive. Reducing calories is likely to leave you chronically tired and even unable to complete a workout. That's certainly not good for your VO_2max.

Reducing your bike's weight is certainly a possibility. That usually comes down to money. As you are undoubtedly aware, lighter bike equipment costs more. And with the way today's high-end bikes are built, you're unlikely to reduce weight by more than a few ounces, which is insignificant even on uphills. It's better just to focus on getting in better shape through training.

So, how can you improve aerobic capacity with training? There are two broad categories of training that will achieve this. The first is training volume—sometimes called "saddle time." This is the most basic of the two. Simply put in a lot more miles or hours every week and your aerobic capacity will increase. Your body will become better at processing oxygen. But this will only take you so far. To top off your aerobic capacity, you'll need to perform high-intensity interval training. Doing workouts that include 4-minute and shorter efforts at a very high intensity—well above your anaerobic threshold (to be explained shortly)—with brief recoveries after each will improve your body's capacity for processing oxygen. Most riders equate this with their lung capacity, but that's only part of the story. It also involves your heart, veins, muscles, and body chemistry. All are improved by doing these very hard interval workouts. (See "Anaerobic Endurance Main Sets" in the appendix for details.)

I should warn you at this point that if you have not been doing such intervals, you must start conservatively. A couple of 30-second high-intensity intervals with 30 seconds of recovery after each is a safe way to start. Notice I said "a couple"—not a dozen or more. Then gradually, over several weeks, increase the durations of the hard efforts until you can do several high-effort intervals in the 2- to 4-minute range with equal or somewhat briefer recoveries after each. In Chapter 8 we'll explain how to get started with intervals if you've not done such training before or if it's been a long time since you have.

Serious riders combine both of these workout types—high volume and high-intensity intervals—into their training seasons. We'll return to this topic in Chapter 7, when we discuss planning your season.

ANAEROBIC THRESHOLD

This fitness marker brings us right back to oxygen. You've probably seen an athlete being tested in a lab or clinic with a plastic mask over their nose and mouth while riding a bike or running on a treadmill. You may have done this yourself. The test is measuring oxygen utilization. Its purpose is usually to determine the athlete's VO_2max, but it also discovers the athlete's anaerobic threshold along the way. The mask is hooked up to a device that measures the oxygen being breathed in and out during the test. At the very end of this "graded exercise test," when the athlete is at maximal effort, the volume of oxygen being processed is measured. This happens right before exhaustion, which is when VO_2max is achieved. But before getting to the final, high end of oxygen consumption, the athlete passes through what is called the anaerobic threshold. This is the intensity level at which, as the workload gets harder, the body gradually switches over from using both carbohydrate and fat for fuel to only carbohydrate. The anaerobic threshold is marked by a heavily increased breathing cycle as the demand for oxygen greatly increases.

On a scale of 0 to 10, 10 being the greatest exertion or effort, the anaerobic threshold is about 7 whereas aerobic capacity is 10. (This scale is sometimes referred to as a rating of perceived exertion, or RPE; see a full explanation in Chapter 6.) So, the anaerobic threshold is certainly a high level of effort, but not nearly as high as an effort at VO_2max.

This level of exertion, at approximately 7 out of 10, is also referred to as "lactate threshold" and "functional threshold." The names simply indicate how the threshold was determined. While the anaerobic threshold test involves measuring oxygen, the lactate threshold is determined by measuring, you guessed it, lactate—a product of carbohydrate consumption. As you pedal harder against a resistance, you'll produce more lactate. The functional threshold is determined by using a field test, which is much less expensive than going to a lab or clinic to be tested. In fact, it's free. We'll return to the concept of functional threshold several times in the following chapters because it's a cheap—but by no means easy—way of determining your threshold.

A higher anaerobic threshold, as a percentage of your aerobic capacity, means you are more fit. An extremely fit rider may have a threshold that is 75 to 85 percent of his or her VO_2max. A beginner's anaerobic threshold may only be around 60 percent. The higher the percentage, the faster you can ride before you reach your anaerobic threshold.

The ceiling for your aerobic capacity is largely determined by heredity. In contrast, your threshold as a percentage is strictly a result of training. Long intervals done at or near your anaerobic threshold bring significant improvements. In the workouts appendix, you will find a category of workouts called "Muscular Endurance." These focus on improving your anaerobic threshold. Another category of training called "Anaerobic Endurance" focuses on improving the amount of work you can do once you exceed your anaerobic threshold.

ECONOMY

The third marker of endurance fitness is economy. You are probably aware of the concept because of your car's "economy rating." Some cars get a lot of miles per gallon (or kilometers per liter) of fuel while others don't. When a car can cover more distance per unit of energy, it's more economical. Cycling, and exercise in general, is no different. Some people are very economical, and others aren't. The amount of energy you expend while riding at any given intensity determines how economical you are. The greater your economy, the greater your fitness.

Although you are certainly expending fuel while pedaling, you don't have a fuel gauge as on your car. So, how is economy determined in cycling? This question brings us back once again to oxygen. It takes oxygen to convert carbohydrate and fat into energy. As your energy expenditure increases, oxygen consumption also increases. All we have to do then is determine the oxygen taken in during exercise in order to measure energy expenditure.

This is done using the same test method described earlier for aerobic capacity, with the mask over the nose and mouth hooked up to an oxygen-measuring device. The test method is pretty simple. The technician has the rider warm up and then ride at a given intensity (this usually involves a power meter) for a set period of time—generally a few minutes. If, over the several weeks between such tests, the amount of oxygen consumed at this standard intensity decreases, then the athlete is becoming more economical. Less fuel is needed to pedal at a fixed intensity for a fixed amount of time. Pretty simple, or so it seems.

How do you improve economy with training? That's where the fun begins, because there are several physiological determinants of how much oxygen you consume while riding and therefore your economy. Some are set by genetics and can't be changed. Let's start with those over which you have no control.

Every cyclist has a unique physical makeup inherited from his or her parents that affects fuel usage. For example, research has shown that having a long thigh bone relative to total leg length is beneficial for economy in cycling. You're not going to change that. There are others in this category, such as the width of your shoulders. Narrow shoulders are beneficial when time trialing outdoors because they create less aerodynamic drag than wide shoulders. Drag is a huge energy robber. The list of these physical economy determinants over which you have no control goes on and on. Although it's not useful to dwell on them because they can't be changed, it is interesting to note that most e-racing apps standardize drag based on rider height and weight, so the individual advantages or disadvantages you have outdoors may not help or hurt you as much indoors.

Some physical aspects of pedaling a bike, over which you have a bit of control, also affect economy. For example, a greater concentration of slow-twitch muscle fibers in cycling-specific muscles will help you waste less energy. Endurance training has been shown to produce some limited benefits in this area. A lack of flexibility around the hips (especially tightness in the lower back and hamstrings) limits how aerodynamically you can position yourself on a bike and therefore affects how much energy is needed to overcome drag. But with some focused stretching, you *may* be able to improve that a bit and become more flexible and therefore more economical.

The third category of your physical makeup that greatly affects economy and over which you have a great deal of control is cycling skills—especially pedaling skills. Many riders seem unaware there is skill associated with pedaling. But there is. And quite a bit. By improving your pedaling skills you can become much more economical and therefore more fit. That, of course, means you go faster.

The most important pedaling skill has to do with how early in the stroke you start to apply a downward force to the pedal. You're probably familiar with the observation that novice riders often pedal in "squares" while experienced riders have a more circular stroke. This simply comes down to when and for how long force is applied to the pedal. If you start to push earlier in the downstroke and continue that downward push longer through the stroke, your pedaling becomes more circular and therefore more economical.

For workouts that focus especially on pedaling to improve your economy see the "Speed Skills" workouts in the appendix.

Other skills influence economy too, such as how well you corner, your comfortable cadence ranges under various conditions, and your mechanics for sprinting and climbing hills. We could even include how skilled a road cyclist is at staying out of the wind with tactical drafting. All of these, of course, also save energy.

Other training factors can also improve your economy. One of the most common among serious riders is strength training. Crosstraining is an important part of performance. By becoming stronger and therefore more powerful, you also become more economical. You can ride faster given the same energy expenditure. But you need to be careful with this one because significantly increasing your body mass is likely to slow you down when climbing.

THE INTERACTION OF BIKE AND RIDER WHEN INDOORS

When riding indoors as compared to on the road, you have probably noticed some differences in how your body moves, in your physical response, or in the effort needed to turn the pedals. Most of these differences relate very closely to economy—and, of course, to the fact that you are not moving forward. Because of these differences, aerobic capacity and anaerobic threshold are also affected. Peak performance in each of the three physiological fitness markers explained earlier does not happen in isolation from the other two. If your economy is reduced for some reason, your aerobic capacity will decrease—as will your anaerobic threshold. Economy plays a key role in how fit you are. And it is the fitness marker that varies the most when riding indoors. Let's look at how economy changes when you ride inside and what can be done about it.

HEAT

One of the most common misconceptions about exercising indoors is that you're exercising harder than outdoors because you're sweating more heavily. Sweating profusely does not quite indicate greater exercise intensity, though. And, in fact, the excess heat that you must deal with indoors is a common economy robber. When you are outside on the road and riding along at a brisk pace, a lot of air flows over your body, cooling you down. Indoors, there is none. You're not moving. This results in heat accumulation, which causes the body to work harder to cool itself by shunting blood away from the muscles and to the skin. It's similar to the way a car's air conditioner uses energy and reduces gas mileage. You have to work harder. There isn't enough blood to meet all of your body's needs. You're also sweating heavily, thereby losing fluids, causing your blood to become thicker. Both of these changes result in a higher heart rate at a given speed or power. And your breathing is also heavier. Through all of these changes, energy is being wasted as far as your muscles are concerned. Fortunately, there's a simple solution to the heating problem: By setting up one or more fans while riding indoors, you can more closely simulate the cooling effect of outdoor riding. Problem solved.

BODY AND BIKE MOVEMENT

The next common robber of energy has to do with the mechanical interaction between you and the bike. As we have said, the indoor trainer does not move; but what does that really mean? An outdoor bicycle frame is built to flex with the rider in three ways: vertically, laterally (torsion), and at the bottom bracket/drivetrain, and they relate to each other. Let's have a look at how the three types of flex influence what you feel out on the road and how that differs inside.

Vertical Flex

Road bikes will offer a smooth ride when the frame is designed with the right amount of vertical flex. This ride quality is largely due to increased road compliance (the nature of contact between the tires and the road), which ultimately leads to better control and handling. If the frame is too stiff, the rider will notice that the handling suffers as the tires lose contact with the road surface, even if just for a split second. The rider then has less control over direction and speed. When brought indoors and set on a trainer, your outdoor bike has the same vertical flex, but because the bike isn't responding to the contours of a road, vertical flex of an outdoor bike doesn't occur nearly as much.

Indoor cycles, in comparison, are built with nearly no vertical flex. This lack of vertical flex can contribute to an improved economy because you are transferring more downward force to the pedal in the absence of the "bounce" effect of vertical oscillation.

Lateral/Torsional Flex

Torsional flex occurs when the head tube twists in relation to the seat tube, shifting their orientation onto different planes. All frames have torsional flex regardless of frame material or quality. Would you like to see torsional flex for yourself? Straddle your bike while standing in front of a mirror. When facing the mirror, push your hands to the left and your butt to the right without moving your feet. The twisting that you are seeing is torsional flex. As with vertical flex, the torsional flex of your road bicycle will occur also when it's used on an indoor stationary trainer. But there is no torsional flex in an indoor, stand-alone cycling machine. This lack of torsional flex on an indoor cycle can actually help to improve economy as no energy used to drive the pedals down is lost due to torsional flex absorbing it.

Bottom Bracket/Drivetrain

This is the most talked about and least understood of the three forms of flex. Is a stiffer frame really better? Does a bottom bracket flex truly result in inefficiency and a loss of energy? I contend that the opposite is true because a small amount of bottom bracket flex acts as a spring that can store some of your pedaling energy and return it to the drivetrain. Of course, it's also possible that this lateral flex can be excessive, which wastes energy. With each downward push on the pedal, the rider is also pushing sideways because the pedal is positioned to the side of the bike rather than on the centerline.

This sideways force flexes the frame until the lateral tension is released. In terms of the pedal stroke, the bottom bracket begins its sideways movement at the top of the pedal stroke and then releases at the bottom of the stroke when we unweight the leg. The flexing and return acts as a spring that stores and releases the lateral energy. This flex and return smooths out the power transmission to the ground by helping you have a more even transfer of power, which also improves road compliance. The bottom bracket flex of your bicycle on a trainer occurs just as it does outdoors; there is no bottom bracket flex in an indoor cycle. This lack of bottom bracket flex on a dedicated indoor cycle will reduce your indoor riding economy.

Stabilization

In addition to frame flex, when you ride on the road the bike alternately rocks, or oscillates, side to side. This is magnified when sprinting. The rocking is due to the push-pull movement of your core muscles in stabilizing the body while driving the pedals at a high force. While the bike has a slight sway even when not sprinting, your upper body is relatively still. It's just the opposite when your bike is locked into a stationary trainer. The bike doesn't move, but your body sways a bit. If most of your riding is done on the road, you've become economically adapted to having a quiet upper body and a swaying bike. Whenever you change something that you had been adapted to, economy suffers because you're using slightly different muscles than when on the road. The good news is that after a couple of weeks of indoor riding, this will become the norm, and you won't waste as much energy—you'll become more economical at riding indoors. While you won't become adapted to out-of-the-saddle, max-effort sprinting with your road bike on an indoor trainer, you can improve your form for max-effort seated sprints and accelerations.

PEDALING SKILLS

Of all the indoor energy robbers, the most common is poor pedaling form. The type of indoor equipment you use can significantly change your pedaling compared to what it is like on the road, and it can result in a significant decrease in power output. Pedaling skills have a lot to do with the dead spot in your pedal stroke. This occurs when the pedals are at the 12 and 6 o'clock positions. When pedaling, you come to this position twice in every cycle, or about 10,000 times per hour. During this brief but frequent interlude, while riding outdoors on flat terrain, the rear wheel continues to rotate because of momentum. But on some trainers—especially rollers and older wind-resistance, fluid, and magnetic trainers—the rear wheel immediately slows down when the pedals are in the dead spot since there is no tension on the chain. It's not a substantial slowdown, but it's enough to waste energy because you have to apply a great deal more force on every stroke to maintain the power and speed of the rear wheel. And that's happening about 10,000 times per hour, making for a lot of wasted energy. For some riders on some trainers, it could amount to a 10 to 15 percent reduction in economy.

If your indoor training machine has a flywheel, you're much less likely to see any change in economy when indoors versus outdoors (see Chapter 3 for details on indoor training equipment). The weight of the flywheel boosts the momentum of the rear wheel so it behaves more like it does when on the road.

If you don't have a flywheel, over time your pedaling technique will adapt and slightly correct how you pedal. This could take a few weeks. In the meantime, your training is less effective. But it's possible to speed up the adaptation by consciously adjusting how you pedal when indoors. The good news is that this new adapted pedaling technique will also improve your road riding economy.

So, how do you change your pedaling technique? Let's go back to the square-pedaling novice and the circular-pedaling experienced rider. The novice starts applying a downward force to the pedal at slightly before the 3 o'clock position. And it ends very quickly at around 4 o'clock or even sooner. The rest of the pedal stroke is usually also wasteful as the novice typically lets his or her foot rest on the pedal except for that very brief episode of force application. The "recovering" leg resting on the pedal simply means that the other leg has to work very hard, for a very short period of time, to keep the pedals turning and maintain speed or power. That's a huge waste of energy.

The experienced rider, however, applies force on the downstroke very early—at about 1 o'clock. And force is applied all the way down to about 5 o'clock. He or she also doesn't let the recovering leg "go to sleep" on the backside of the stroke. Nor does the economical rider pull up on the pedal, as many people think they do (the exception is when sprinting). This would also be very wasteful and result in extreme fatigue in the hip flexor muscles within a few minutes. The experienced rider simply unweights the pedal on the upstroke (from 6 to 12 o'clock).

If this circular pedaling technique is new to you or you feel it could be improved, how do you make the changes in order to be more economical? As mentioned earlier, there are workouts under the heading "Speed Skills Main Sets" in the appendix. These will help you refine your pedaling skills. But we'll also explain here how you can go about changing your pedaling technique so that you are more economical both indoors and on the road.

Note, again, that this is not just a change for your indoor pedaling. It is intended to be applied both indoors and outdoors, and on flat terrain and hills. In fact, you'll probably discover that you climb better once you master this pedaling technique.

Let's start by looking at the downstroke. Remember that the goal is to start the force application to the pedal early in the stroke—at around 1 o'clock. The key to doing this is your heel. As you pass through 12 o'clock, the heel should be lowered a little so that it's level with the ball of the foot, or even a bit below it, by 1 o'clock. This will allow you to drive the pedal slightly forward and slightly downward at the same time. As the foot approaches the 5 o'clock position the heel is raised somewhat so that it is just above the ball of the foot. This may only be about one-half inch or a centimeter. The foot position is maintained all the way through the backstroke. And then, as mentioned before, you should feel like you are taking weight off of the pedal—but not pulling up on it. The slightly raised heel will help you do this.

Let us toss in a caveat here. If you are a triathlete or time trialist who rides a very upright bike, with the seat tube at about 76 degrees or steeper, you will find it very difficult to get your heel below or even perhaps level with the ball of the foot when seated on the saddle. That's normal for this type of bike because your seat is positioned farther forward relative to the bottom bracket. Just get your heel as low as you can get it at 1 o'clock without putting undo stress on the calf muscle or ankle.

INDOOR "CLIMBING"

Indoors, there is no way to simulate the uphill fight against gravity. And gravity has a big effect on how you pedal and interact with the bike, especially outdoors. On the road when climbing a hill, as soon as you get to the dead spot in your pedal stroke the bike starts to slow down significantly due to gravity. This is actually quite similar to what you experience on an indoor trainer that doesn't have a flywheel. So, you might say that riding a trainer without a flywheel is like you're always climbing. About the only way to improve on this and more closely simulate a hill is to raise the front wheel slightly to mimic the angle of the bike when climbing. Some indoor cycling equipment, such as the Wahoo KICKR Climb and the Wahoo KICKR Smart Bike, can automatically adjust your climbing angle based on input from an app. When climbing a relatively steep hill outdoors, lowering your heel and applying force earlier in the pedal stroke is beneficial. While it won't be the same thing as climbing on the road, you can get close indoors by sitting upright, shifting back in the saddle, and slightly lowering your heel as your foot crosses the top of the stroke.

INDOOR "DRAG"

When riding indoors, you also can't simulate drag—the resistive flow of air over your body when riding fast. But if you're a triathlete or time trialist, you can certainly continue to practice riding in a more aerodynamic position, as if you were riding into the wind. Such a position typically involves being a bit forward on the saddle with your head in the "turtle" position and your arms in close to the body. In this posture it can be a bit difficult to get your heel low, especially when riding a steep frame, but continue trying to refine this pedaling method to improve your speed when back on the road, where you'll be facing the wind once again.

INDOOR CYCLING EQUIPMENT

The challenge in presenting a chapter on indoor cycling equipment is that the marketplace changes quickly, and the pace is only accelerating. Going into exhaustive detail about the features of specific models of indoor trainers, indoor cycles, and apps would make this chapter obsolete before the book ever reached your hands. Although the bells and whistles offered on indoor cycling equipment change quickly, the underlying functionalities are far more consistent. While you don't have to know all the details about how the equipment works, it is helpful to know about the several ways you can ride inside, and their opportunities and limitations. Investing in the equipment that best meets your goals and requirements will help you enjoy riding inside, which means you will want to do it more often.

TRADITIONAL INDOOR CYCLING EQUIPMENT

I am a big fan of technology that makes training more efficient and precise. After all, my son Dirk, friend Gear Fisher, and I worked together on the development of TrainingPeaks software, which was one of the first online tools that allowed athletes and coaches to upload and synthesize training data from a wide range of tools, like heart rate monitors, power meters, and GPS units. Yet, while athletes and coaches now generate and have access to more data than ever before, I also recognize that athletes can achieve great progress by applying sound sports science to uncomplicated workouts performed with basic equipment. In fact, there can be some advantages to using old-school indoor cycling equipment.

REAR-WHEEL STATIONARY TRAINERS

The starting point for riding inside is mounting your personal bicycle to a stationary trainer that secures the bike by clamping down on the rear axle or quick release. The resistance you are pedaling against comes from an open fan, magnets, or an enclosed fan spinning in oil. These resistance units are connected to a metal roller that gets pressed against the rear tire of your bicycle. As you produce power with your legs and lungs to turn your rear wheel, the metal roller turns and engages the resistance unit.

With wind and fluid trainers, fans turn in air or oil to create resistance that increases exponentially as you increase your effort level. This is similar to the way air resistance increases as you go faster outdoors; accelerating from 10 miles per hour to 15 miles per hour is a lot easier than accelerating from 25 to 30 miles per hour. At 10 miles per hour, about half your power output is used to punch a hole in the air. And at 30 miles per hour outdoors on a windless day, up to 90 percent of a cyclist's power output goes to overcoming air resistance.

Manufacturers design wind and fluid trainers to have resistance curves that mirror outdoor conditions, and then they pair the resistance unit with a sizable flywheel that helps replicate the forward momentum you have outdoors. Without the flywheel, your rear wheel would slow down too quickly when you reduce pressure on the pedals, almost like you slammed on the brakes while on the road. The interplay between the resistance unit and the flywheel creates a trainer's realistic "road feel," or how similar changes in effort translate to changes in resistance compared to being outdoors. The most notable difference between wind and fluid trainers is that wind trainers are the most economical option and fluid trainers are orders of magnitude quieter.

Magnetic resistance trainers work by spinning a metal disk in a magnetic field. The primary difference between "mag" trainers and wind or fluid versions is that the resistance increases linearly or can be set at constant levels, depending on the model. On the positive side, mag trainers are quieter than wind trainers and are useful for maintaining a constant resistance. However, one of the biggest drawbacks to magnetic resistance at specific levels is that a rider can overcome the resistance by building up enough speed that the flywheel's momentum effectively reduces the power the rider needs to contribute to keep going. While mag trainers can be less expensive than other options, the linear increase in resistance provides a less realistic simulation of real-world training.

ROLLERS

One of the oldest ways to ride inside, riding rollers requires a rider to balance on parallel metal cylinders connected by an elastic band. As the rear wheel rotates one of the rear rollers, the band rotates the front roller, which in turn rotates the front wheel. With nothing holding the bicycle upright, angular momentum from the wheels allows the rider to maintain balance. Becoming proficient at riding rollers requires practice, and riding rollers requires more attention and focus than riding a stationary trainer or dedicated indoor cycle. While this makes many riders shy away from rollers, they can be useful for improving performance.

By amplifying small side-to-side movements and choppy pedal strokes, rollers help riders smooth out their pedaling mechanics and adopt a "quiet" riding style. (Recall the discussion on pedaling skills in Chapter 2.) On a stationary trainer you can thrash your body from side to side or jump on the pedals out of the saddle. On rollers those actions will send you careening sideways to a rapid and unpleasant stop. Other times it's not the effort that gets you in trouble. Getting too drawn into your training data or letting your mind drift can result in a physical drift that also sends you off the side of the rollers. On the other hand, reaching for a water bottle, a towel to wipe sweat off your brow, or the remote to change the channel adds an element of skill and stability that transfers well to outdoor riding. If you can smoothly take a drink or ride with one hand—or no hands—on rollers, you'll improve your ability to maintain a straight line in the same circumstances outdoors.

The increased engagement and focus required to stay upright is part of what appeals to roller aficionados. Just like the real-world outdoors, you can't simply turn your brain off and pedal. This makes rollers a great option for staying engaged during long endurance rides indoors or moderate-intensity interval workouts. For high-intensity intervals and sprint workouts, the balance requirement for rollers can create an impediment to high-quality training. When I prescribe interval workouts with maximum power efforts for 40 seconds, separated by only 20 seconds of recovery, the goal is for you to repeatedly produce the highest power output you can for 15 or 20 efforts. When you have to reserve part of your mental and physical effort for maintaining your balance on rollers, it takes away from the effectiveness of the workout.

Resistance on rollers can come from the diameter of the cylinders (small-diameter rollers naturally create more resistance than large-diameter rollers) or a resistance unit tethered to one of the rollers. And although rollers have traditionally been the most analog of indoor cycling options, the connected technologies featured in smart trainers are making their way to rollers as well.

ADVANTAGES OF TRADITIONAL INDOOR CYCLING EQUIPMENT

Rear-wheel trainers and rollers may seem like antiquated technology compared to smart trainer options and internet-connected indoor cycles, but they have some significant advantages.

No Electricity Needed

The critical limitation for smart trainers is that most have to be plugged in. This is particularly problematic when it comes to using a trainer for a prerace warm-up. Whether you are getting ready for a criterium, cyclocross race, cross-country mountain bike event, or triathlon, your warm-up options are often limited to riding around on local roads or setting up a trainer or rollers in a parking lot. The trainer offers the opportunity for a more controlled and predictable warm-up, keeps you in close proximity to your gear and clothing, and eliminates the risks of getting lost, having a mechanical, or getting hit by a car.

Easy Setup

As I'll explain soon, there are great features of and benefits to using a smart trainer, but there is also a hassle involved in connecting all the devices. Once you get your setup dialed in, the time and labor required definitely diminish, but the simplicity of non-connected trainers and rollers can be viewed as a positive. If you have a plan for your workout and you're going to control your intensity by perceived exertion, heart rate, or a bicycle-mounted power meter, you don't necessarily need to add the complications of connecting to apps and the internet to go for a bike ride.

Developing Internal Motivation

The most important advantage of using "analog" trainers is that you have to call upon your own motivation to achieve the desired intensity level. Smart trainers have an ergometer mode (discussed in the next section), which a lot of athletes use for structured workouts because the trainer controls the resistance, and all they have to do is pedal. Let's say you have a workout that is 12 one-minute intervals at 450 watts, separated by one minute of easy spinning recovery at 150 watts. With ergometer mode, when each interval starts, the resistance increases to 450 watts and stays there for a minute, then drops to 150 watts, and so on. I'll talk more about "erg" mode later in this chapter when I go into more depth on smart trainers, but the point I want to make here is that when you train outdoors or with an analog trainer, you need to find the internal motivation to produce 450 watts for a minute and repeat it 11 more times. In competition you have to dig deep to produce the power for a race-winning attack and hold it long enough to reach the finish line. You can develop fitness and power in erg mode, but when put to the test in the real world, some athletes realize they haven't developed the mental fortitude to access and apply that power on command. In Chapter 9 I'll offer more guidance on pairing workouts with the most suitable trainer technology choices.

SMART TRAINERS

The concept behind smart trainers existed for many years in physiology labs before the technology became available to consumers. When we ran lactate threshold and VO$_2$max tests in a lab setting, we used an ergometer—an indoor cycle whose resistance was controlled by a computer. During a classic ramp test, the computer would start with a resistance whereby riders had to produce 150 watts to match it; every 4 minutes, the required power output ticked up by 50 watts. That same concept drives the modern-day smart trainers that are available to any athlete wanting to train indoors: A computer—with which the rider can interact—controls the resistance.

HOW SMART TRAINERS WORK

While one of the benefits of a traditional trainer is that it is self-contained, most smart trainers are useless without a number of other components. If you're going to use a smart trainer, you will need the following:

- **The smart trainer itself, naturally.** Most smart trainers feature direct drive, which replaces the rear wheel with a cassette mounted directly to the trainer. There are a few direct drive fluid resistance trainers, but this feature is mostly reserved for smart trainers.

- **A power source.** Smart trainers use electromagnets to smoothly adjust the resistance you feel as you ride. Increasing electrical current increases the drag the magnets apply to the trainer's metal flywheel. When the electrical current drops, there is less drag on the flywheel, and pedaling gets easier. The vast majority of smart trainers need to be plugged in to an electrical outlet to function. There are a few that are "self-powered," meaning you generate electrical power as you pedal, and that power is used to adjust the resistance. This is good if you want to use the trainer in a parking lot to warm up before a race, but it also means you have to be pedaling in order to pair the trainer to apps and other devices.

THE SMART TRAINER'S ORIGIN STORY

Once the idea of computer-controlled resistance spread beyond the exercise physiology lab, the next step in development was to attach an electrically controlled resistance unit to a rear-wheel trainer and hook it up to a computer that could control the trainer. RacerMate, which commercialized the first wind-resistance trainer in 1975, developed the first commercially available smart trainer in 1986. Its CompuTrainer used electromagnets to vary the resistance applied to the friction roller on a rear-wheel trainer. That opened up a whole new world of opportunities for indoor cycling. With a CompuTrainer you could have an ergometer mode and create structured interval workouts, or you could use data from real road courses to simulate the hills and undulations of that course indoors. Later you could connect several CompuTrainers together so cyclists could race each other or participate in group training classes.

CompuTrainer was the gold standard for electronic indoor trainers throughout the 1990s and well into the 2000s. They were so well built that they had remarkable accuracy and repeatability, meaning that a 200-watt effort today was the same as a 200-watt effort tomorrow. They were sturdy and durable and—at the time—generated more training data than any bicycle-mounted power meter. But as sometimes happens with pioneering products, new technologies emerged that enabled competitors to innovate faster and eliminate some of the barriers that prevented CompuTrainer from reaching widespread adoption.

As the story goes, engineer and boat-dock builder Chip Hawkins was also a triathlete who liked using a CompuTrainer. What he didn't like was that CompuTrainer was a closed system, meaning you had to use its proprietary software and controller to go for a ride. He wanted a different controller, and he went as far as designing it himself and offering it to RacerMate. When they declined to work with Chip, he had the idea to create the trainer and controller he wanted, which led to the development of the Wahoo KICKR.

The first Wahoo KICKR debuted in 2012. The KICKR feature that sparked a major disruption in the trainer world was its open platform. When I worked on the development of TrainingPeaks, one of the first principles we established was that the software had to be agnostic, meaning we wanted to support uploads of training data from any brand of device and wanted coaches to be able to write their own workouts and apply their own training philosophies. Wahoo did the same with smart trainers, allowing cyclists and   >>>

Continued

triathletes to use the Wahoo Fitness app or record data to a Garmin or other head unit. The data, in turn, could be exported to a number of training software options. Eventually, the trainer itself could be controlled by a variety of apps operating from a phone, laptop, or Apple TV.

Although the Wahoo KICKR was relatively expensive (about $1,200 compared to a $250 fluid trainer), it was the right product at the right time. Power meters on bikes, and the idea of training with power, had become ubiquitous by the late 2000s. Smartphones and apps had arrived with the launch of the first iPhone in 2007. And more specific to cycling technology, power meters and cycling computers started using Bluetooth to connect and transfer information. (Previously, training devices like power meters, heart rate monitors, and speed and cadence sensors communicated with watches and cycling computers only via an ANT+ signal. While ANT+ worked well and is still used, Bluetooth connectivity was the standard in phones and laptops, whereas connecting a device to a phone or laptop via ANT+ required a special dongle.) All of these factors converged to help athletes see the value smart trainers provided, and to make smart trainers easy to use and convenient to connect wirelessly. Within a few short years, every major indoor cycling brand put a smart trainer on the market and, although they were ahead of their time and made a great product, RacerMate failed to adapt to the changes in the market and stopped production of the CompuTrainer in 2017.

- **A controller.** Something has to tell the smart trainer what to do. The two primary ways to control a smart trainer are through an app or with a handlebar-mounted cycling computer that can communicate with the trainer via Bluetooth or ANT+.

- **A connection.** An internet connection may not always be necessary to work a smart trainer, but even if you use the trainer offline, a data connection will be necessary for uploading your training data to a fitness tracker. Having an internet connection allows you to use more features, including virtual group rides and e-racing.

One of the reasons a smart trainer is so versatile is that you can set it up to operate like a magnetic trainer, a wind/fluid trainer, or an ergometer. The modes available depend on the trainer and/or app you are using but fall into the following categories.

LEVEL OR FLUID MODE

In level mode, which is sometimes called fluid mode, your smart trainer acts like a fluid resistance trainer. As you ride faster, the resistance ramps up according to a preset power curve designed to replicate the experience on a wind or fluid trainer. When controlling a smart trainer with an app, however, you can typically adjust the power curve to change the resistance at a given speed. This is useful when you want to change the gearing you're using while riding the trainer. If you adjust the power curve to be lighter/lower, you will be using bigger gears and turning the flywheel (via the rear wheel or cassette) faster. This leads to greater momentum, like you're pedaling on flat ground at high speed. If you adjust the power curve to be heavier/higher, you'll experience more resistance at lower speeds and be using smaller gears. You'll have less momentum, meaning the flywheel will slow more quickly in response to even small dips in power output. This will feel more like climbing a steep hill, where you experience a slight deceleration between each pedal stroke.

When to Use Level Mode

Some smart trainers default to this mode when the trainer is plugged in to a power source but is not connected to a cycling computer or app. While this at least lets you do something with the trainer, it is becoming increasingly rare that a person has access to electrical power but doesn't have access to at least a phone app.

The primary benefit to using this mode is that you have to control the power output and effort level yourself, just like you do out on the road or trail. If your workout calls for holding 300 watts for 20 minutes, you will have to bring your output up to that level and—more importantly—hold it there yourself. If you lose focus, your power drops, and you have to work to get back up to your target power. If you drive it too hard, the resistance increases and pushes you over your target power. This might not seem like much of a problem unless you are riding at the limit of your sustainable power. Pushing 10 percent over that target power for too long is likely to cause excessive fatigue and require you to reduce your power output before the end of the interval.

RESISTANCE OR BRAKE MODE

If a smart trainer has a resistance or brake mode, it means the resistance will increase linearly with speed. This is essentially a way to replicate the friction-based resistance from indoor cycles that use brake pads or a belt to create friction against the flywheel. On those bikes, the tighter you turn the resistance knob, the more friction is applied to the flywheel. On a smart trainer, this mode is often represented as a percentage, from 0 to 100 percent resistance. Because this is the least similar to the way cyclists experience changes in resistance during outdoor cycling, this mode is not used very much on smart trainers.

ERG MODE

When you use erg (ergometer) mode, the trainer's resistance is controlled by an external source, either an app or a cycling computer. Let's say your workout for the day calls for three 20-minute efforts at 250 watts, separated by 10 minutes of easy spinning at 125 watts. Using erg mode, the trainer will try to keep the resistance at 250 watts during the intervals, no matter the cadence or gearing you are using. And when an interval is over, the trainer will automatically lower the tension and set your target power to 125 watts.

Some apps and cycling computers also allow you to adjust the target power manually, meaning you can notch your target power up and down incrementally whenever you want. This can be useful if want to use erg mode but don't have access to a prebuilt workout. However, it is more convenient for prolonged intervals and moderate intensities because you have the time to make adjustments. It is difficult to accurately and quickly change power output from 150 to 400 watts for a 60-second interval, and then it's even harder to release the tension at the end of the interval when your legs are screaming and you're cross-eyed and panting uncontrollably.

Shifting gears doesn't do you much good when you are in erg mode, because the trainer will quickly react to keep the resistance constant. The one factor you truly have control over in erg mode is your cadence. Mathematically speaking, power output is the product of force and angular velocity (cadence), which means there is an inverse relationship between force and cadence. If you begin riding an interval at a cadence of 90 rpm and increase it to 100 rpm, to keep the power output at 250 watts, the trainer will reduce the resistance so the force you have to apply to the pedals decreases. On the other hand, if you drop your cadence from 90 to 70 rpm, the trainer ramps up the resistance because you need to use more force to produce 250 watts at a slower cadence.

When to Use Erg Mode

From a training perspective, erg mode is very useful for executing structured interval workouts. Using online training tools, cyclists can build and download workout files that define exactly when and how much the target power output should change. You can use structured workouts with or without erg mode. When you use them without erg mode, you will get a notification that it is time to increase or decrease your power output, but it will be up to you to respond. When you combine a structured workout with erg mode, you essentially hit "start" at the beginning of the workout and let the smart trainer control the changes in resistance automatically.

Erg mode offers athletes and coaches an unprecedented level of accuracy because the duration and intensity of intervals and recovery periods are preset. You can't quit an interval 30 seconds early or take an extra minute of recovery between hard efforts. This lets an athlete focus on producing the power rather than keeping track of the interval count.

High-intensity interval workouts are perhaps the best application for erg mode because they involve a high number of short intervals separated by short recovery periods. During repeated hard efforts without erg mode, athletes lose track of what interval they're on and have trouble watching a timer. When I want an athlete to dig really deep, the safest and most effective environment for those workouts is indoors with erg mode. In the last 30 seconds of a 3-minute maximum effort, a rider can put their head down, close their eyes, and completely drain themselves to the point that they slump over the bars and gasp for breath when it's over. For obvious reasons, that would be dangerous and irresponsible on the road, track, or trail.

When Erg Mode Defeats You

Erg mode is an unforgiving taskmaster. If you are in the middle of a particularly challenging workout, you might start struggling to maintain your target power output, and your cadence will drop. The trainer doesn't know or care that you are struggling. All it knows is that when cadence drops, resistance must increase in order to keep the target power output steady. So the trainer clamps down harder, making it even more difficult to maintain your cadence. This death spiral continues until the resistance becomes so great that your feet grind to a halt.

Smart trainers and apps handle the death spiral differently, but they are programmed to recognize that you're stuck and then release the tension so you can get your cadence back up to speed. Many of the apps that support structured workouts will release the tension, let you get your cadence back up, and give you an automatic countdown before resetting to the target power for the interval.

The Disadvantages of Erg Mode

Erg mode can make you strong, but it won't make you smart. Excessive reliance on erg mode creates crucial physical and mental skills gaps that can hurt cyclists and triathletes in outdoor competitions. As I've mentioned in the discussions about analog trainers and level mode on a smart trainer, there is a difference between withstanding the effort required to ride at a fixed output of 400 watts for 5 minutes, as set by erg mode, and having the grit and internal motivation to reach and sustain 400 watts for 5 minutes on your own. Similarly, in the last 30 seconds of that 5-minute effort outdoors, you have to keep your head up and maintain control of your bike. On the other end of the spectrum, long-course triathletes and ultra-endurance cyclists have to develop the mental fortitude to maintain their goal pace after several hours on the bike.

The accuracy that makes erg mode so effective for interval training also makes it completely unrealistic compared to cycling outdoors or even with other modes of indoor cycling. Maintaining a fairly steady power output on the road requires constant adjustments to cadence, force, and speed based on undulations in the road and changes in wind and rolling resistance. Learning to manage these variables is essential for success outdoors.

It would seem logical that time trial and long-distance triathlon competitors would go fastest by completing the entire distance at their maximum sustainable power output. In other words, if an elite cyclist can ride at 350 watts for 60 minutes on an ergometer, wouldn't it be fastest to ride at 350 watts from start to finish during a time trial outdoors? No. The fastest way to complete a real-world course is to use more power when it will provide the greatest advantage and use as little power as possible when it makes the least difference. In practice this might mean charging up short hills at 600 watts and coasting in an aerodynamic tuck once the speed reaches 40 mph on a downhill.

ROUTE/SIMULATION MODE

The mode that enabled the explosive growth in indoor cycling is route, or simulation, mode. This mode leverages the electromagnet to seamlessly adjust the resistance based on physical parameters of the rider and the real or virtual route being ridden, including rider weight, cycling position, bike weight, steepness of the terrain, wind speed and direction, and rolling resistance. Typically, you can just input your weight and use presets for the other parameters, but in some systems you can tweak the details to see how those changes could potentially change your pace outdoors.

"Sim" mode is what makes popular route-based apps like Zwift and FulGaz work, as well as virtual group rides and e-racing. With the route data and your weight, the trainer can adjust the resistance to simulate what you would feel if you were actually on a specific course. And based on your power output, the system determines your speed and position on the course relative to other riders.

When to Use Sim Mode

Simulation mode is useful for previewing a real course you will later see in competition. For instance, the Ironman World Championship bike course in Hawaii was one of the first routes created when CompuTrainer was the only smart trainer on the market. Most competitors are only in Hawaii for, at most, a couple of weeks before the race, and many first-time Ironman Kona competitors see the course for the first time the week of the race. Smart trainers gave athletes the opportunity to study the route and plan a pacing strategy based on the terrain. By adjusting variables like bike weight, aerodynamic drag, and wind direction and speed, athletes could also see how equipment changes could affect their speed and how headwinds or crosswinds could impact their pace.

INDOOR CYCLING APPS

In Chapter 5, I talk about the ways we train indoors, some of which involve using apps. Because this chapter is more about indoor cycling equipment itself, I will use this space to talk about the what indoor cycling apps do and how they interact with and connect your other pieces of indoor cycling equipment.

As with discussions of any specific brand of indoor trainer or power meter, indoor cycling apps change so quickly that it doesn't make sense to delve into the features of particular apps in this book. Instead, let's take a look at how to choose apps that best match your goals and training style.

PRIMARY FUNCTIONS

There are three primary functions of an indoor cycling app, and while some apps deliver all three, there are others that only handle one or two. Before you sign up for any of them, consider what you want the app to do.

Record/track data

This is the absolute base-level functionality for a cycling app. However, there are differences between apps in terms of what data they track (physiological stats and ride-specific information, such as terrain and ride speed), whether they can track data themselves or require additional components, and how easily you can access and share that data.

Control your trainer

First you need a smart trainer that can connect to a device or app. Then check to see if the app or device can control the trainer or just accept data from it. Look for trainers, apps, and devices that feature ANT+ FE-C (Fitness Equipment Control) and/or Bluetooth Smart if you want to control a smart trainer from the app or device. Over time, trainer control will become a standard feature on even basic apps and devices, but with the ever-increasing range of combinations, there will inevitably be some that don't play well together.

Connect with other riders

Recording data and controlling a trainer are all you need if you want to train on your own, but apps that allow for social connectivity are some of the most attractive options. These apps open up the possibility for virtual group rides and e-racing (e.g., Zwift), and live group workouts (e.g., Peloton).

ADDITIONAL CONSIDERATIONS

As you shop around for apps and devices, consider these additional aspects of their offerings and how you want to use them.

Subscriptions

When you buy a smart trainer or cycling computer with an indoor cycling mode, there is typically a native app that is free to use with the hardware. The app is often necessary to update the device firmware, configure settings, use the navigation features, and sync workout data to third-party apps.

A paid subscription will be required to use third-party apps that provide content for indoor cycling, including virtual and video routes, structured workouts and training plans, advanced data analytics, and live competitions and workouts. Many athletes switch indoor training apps at some point, or use multiple apps simultaneously, so it is important to have a free or paid subscription to a fitness tracker app, like TrainingPeaks or Strava, so you can sync and save all your training data over time.

The most restrictive scenario is using a device that is only compatible with a proprietary app or that cannot be used without a subscription. In 2020, one example of this is the Peloton bike, which is only compatible with Peloton content, doesn't broadcast data to devices like cycling computers or other apps, and has severely limited functionality in its "free ride" mode.

Device Compatibility and Data Integration

Third-party indoor cycling apps are increasingly agnostic when it comes to device compatibility because they want to allow as many users as possible to use their platform. Nevertheless, confirm that your equipment is compatible with the app of your choice. In most cases, athletes are looking for apps that will work with equipment they already have, and free trials make it easy to try out various apps. If you are just getting started and have your heart set on using a particular app, then it is more important to make sure you are purchasing indoor cycling equipment that's compatible with it. Similarly, the equipment you are using sometimes generates more data than your app can display or track. More isn't always better when it comes to data, but it is important that you have access to data that you want to use.

Offline Availability

Will you need an internet connection to go for a ride inside using your head unit or app of choice? Many head units (Garmin, Wahoo Elemnt, Lezyne, Stages, etc.) and phone-, tablet-, and laptop-based apps can connect to smart trainers through ANT+ and/or Bluetooth and don't require an internet connection to start or record a workout. You will need an internet or cell phone data connection to sync the data to fitness tracking sites, like Strava and TrainingPeaks. Apps that offer streaming content, like Zwift, may not work without an internet connection. Other apps provide the opportunity to download video and workout content while you have an internet connection so you can use it offline. When choosing the apps you want to work with, consider whether you will always have the connectivity required to use them.

INDOOR CYCLES AND SMART BIKES

Instead of using your own bicycle on an indoor trainer, you can ride one of the growing number of dedicated indoor cycles on the market. Indoor cycles have been around for decades, though for many years they were mostly tucked in the corner of hotel gyms or acting as clothing racks in basements. Like indoor trainers, indoor cycles have enjoyed a renaissance in recent years, and the integration of technology into new models makes them an appealing and highly effective addition to a rider's training tool chest. Similarly, newer bikes and improved technology modernized indoor cycling classes, which are now available in cycling studios, like SoulCycle and CycleBar, and presented live, on-demand via Peloton and Echelon. These experiences and communities reinvigorated the indoor cycling industry, which had been overshadowed by other fitness class trends after a boom in the 1990s. More recently, performance cycling companies integrated the app-controlled resistance technology from trainers into indoor cycles to create indoor smart bikes.

INDOOR CYCLES

As with smart trainers and interactive cycling apps, the models and features of specific indoor cycles are evolving too fast for it to be practical to compare individual products in this book. However, it is important for sport-specific cyclists and triathletes to understand some defining characteristics of indoor cycles before deciding which bikes to use in studio classes or purchase for home use.

In order to avoid confusion in the following sections, we need to agree on some terminology. I'm going to use the term "indoor cycle" to broadly encompass the bikes used in studio classes, like SoulCycle and CycleBar, as well as bikes purchased for in-home use from Peloton, Echelon, and Spinning®. While there are important differences within the category of indoor cycles, for sport-specific cyclists and triathletes, I think it's important to make the distinction between indoor cycles and the newer "indoor smart bike." Both categories can be effective for riding inside; it's just that the indoor smart bikes have more in common with smart trainers than with a Peloton or the bikes at your local rec center.

Resistance Design

The earliest indoor cycles used air or friction to create resistance, and they are still available. For the air-resistance models, turning the cranks turns a large fan, which means resistance increases exponentially as you pedal faster. These are useful but very loud, so they are rarely used in studio classes. However, because they are simple, self-contained, and somewhat lighter than indoor cycles that feature big flywheels, air-resistance bikes are more portable and are frequently used on the sidelines of field sports to help athletes warm up.

Friction-based trainers use brake pads or a belt to apply resistance to a heavy flywheel. To increase the resistance, you increase the pressure of the pads or belt against the flywheel. Your power output is determined by the amount of resistance on the flywheel and your cadence (which determines the speed of the flywheel). Unlike air or fluid resistance, which increases exponentially with speed, on a friction-based indoor cycle an increase in flywheel speed (via cadence) leads to a linear increase in resistance. For high-torque, low-cadence efforts, you can tighten the brake pads or belt. On the other end of the spectrum, loosening the pads/belt allows you to get the flywheel moving fast enough that its own momentum can overcome the resistance, meaning minimal power output is required to maintain your cadence and speed.

While air and friction resistance bikes are still available, modern indoor cycles for studio classes and most in-home use feature magnetic resistance.

These bikes have a heavy flywheel that spins between two powerful magnets. The resistance can be increased by moving the magnets closer to the metal flywheel and/or increasing the electrical current to the magnets. However, because the magnets never contact the flywheel, these bikes are far quieter than both air and friction resistance bikes. Magnetic resistance cycles can be made even quieter by using a belt rather than a chain to connect the cranks to the flywheel.

Resistance Control and Measurement

One of the most important distinctions between indoor cycles and smart bikes is how the rider controls the resistance. On an indoor cycle with friction or magnetic resistance, you increase or decrease resistance with a knob, a lever, or buttons. Most studio-based bikes feature a knob; you increase resistance by turning the knob clockwise and decrease it by turning the knob counterclockwise. Magnetic resistance bikes often define resistance by numbered levels, but there is no universally accepted scale. Peloton has 100 levels; others have 32 or 24. And even if bikes have the same number of levels, the resistance that corresponds to a given number is not the same from brand to brand. With friction bikes there are typically no preset levels. While this offers great adjustability, it can make it difficult for riders to precisely repeat efforts.

By and large, the indoor cycles people find in studio classes or use at home do not feature app-controlled resistance like a smart trainer with ANT+ FE-C. This means apps and instructors use a variety of methods for prescribing intensity and leading a class. Many use perceived exertion and cadence, some may use heart rate, and a growing number are using power. Even as more and more classes (in-person and streaming) are based on each rider's individual power zones, it is still up to the rider to adjust the resistance level and cadence to produce the target power. The Stages Cycling indoor cycles have a Stages power meter integrated into the cranks, just like the power meter they produce for outdoor bikes, but it is one of very few indoor cycles that measures power directly. Instead, most calculate power based on the resistance level and cadence, which is generally OK because there are fewer mechanical and environmental variables to account for on an indoor cycle. However, maintenance issues that create additional resistance can lead to lower displayed power outputs for a given effort.

When purchasing an indoor cycle, it is important to determine what training data it records and whether you can share that data with fitness tracking software, like TrainingPeaks or Strava. Similarly, cyclists and triathletes who attend in-person studio classes should determine whether any training data will be available from the classes. If not, you may want to track data independently with a heart rate monitor so you can upload the data afterward.

Adjustability

As a sport-specific cyclist or triathlete, your cycling position plays a critical role in performance. When you are using indoor cycling as a training tool to prepare for outdoor competitions, it is important that you can replicate your competition cycling position indoors. This is one of the key limitations of many indoor cycles used in studios and available for home use. Saddle position is typically micro-adjustable in terms of height, fore-aft, and tilt. And if it's your indoor cycle, you can swap the stock saddle for your favorite shape and width. Other adjustments are not as convenient.

Handlebars. Most indoor cycles feature a proprietary bar shape that offers multiple hand and arm positions, but have few or no options to customize the tilt of the bars or replace them entirely. Handlebar height will be adjustable, although it may have distinct levels rather than fully customized heights. The ability to adjust the fore-aft position of the handlebar (analogous to adjusting the reach on your outdoor bike) is a feature that is harder to find, but for athletes training for outdoor competitions, it is worth the effort or additional cost.

Cranks. For occasional use during an in-person studio class, it's not a big deal that the crank length and Q factor (lateral distance between the pedals) may not be the same as your outdoor bike. If you are purchasing an indoor cycle with the intention of spending many hours on it, these bike-fit parameters may be important to you. Cranks on indoor cycles are typically one-size-fits-all and not adjustable or replaceable.

Pedals. Any pedals that will work on an outdoor bike will work on an indoor cycle, which allows riders to use the same cycling shoes they wear for outdoor rides. If you are going to in-person classes in a cycling studio, you may not have the time or permission to swap pedals at the start of the class, so make sure you have shoes with the correct cleat to match the studio's pedals. You can also participate in classes with non-cycling shoes and flat pedals.

Connectivity and Subscriptions

Peloton's subscription-content model was one of the company's most brilliant and unfortunate decisions. They changed the indoor cycling landscape by streaming live and interactive indoor cycling classes directly to a bike-mounted touchscreen and making that content accessible with a monthly subscription. The unfortunate part is that the bike's functionality is severely limited if you stop the subscription. It functions as a magnetic resistance indoor cycle, but you can't record your ride data or use content from other apps on the bike's large screen. These are all features that could change, but it illustrates the need to understand how dependent your indoor cycle is on apps or online subscriptions.

Many non-Peloton indoor cycles connect to a branded app that can then sync with training apps, or connect directly via Bluetooth or ANT+.

INDOOR SMART BIKES

By maximizing adjustability and precision in training, indoor smart bikes are a better option than indoor cycles for competitive cyclists and triathletes. They combine the micro-adjustability of ergometers you find in professional bike fit studios with the technology and connectivity of smart trainers. Here are some of the features you'll find on indoor smart bikes from companies like Stages Cycling, Wahoo Fitness, Tacx, and Wattbike.

Freewheel Versus Direct Drive

Most indoor cycles for studio or in-home use have a direct drive system similar to a fixed-gear track bike. If the pedals are moving, the flywheel is moving. If the flywheel is moving, your feet have to be moving. This isn't necessarily bad, but athletes training for outdoor cycling have to be aware of the potential for the heavy flywheel's momentum to drive your cadence. If you've ever ridden a fixed-gear bicycle down a hill, you'll remember the sensation of the pedals driving your legs instead of your legs driving the pedals. In contrast, indoor smart bikes use a clutch system that works like the freewheel/cassette on an outdoor bike and allows the rider to coast—another way that indoor smart bikes narrow the gap between riding inside and outside.

Resistance Control and Measurement

Indoor smart bikes feature app- or head-unit-controlled electromagnetic resistance just as smart trainers do. This means you can use similar modes (level, route, ergometer) depending on the training session you want. They use ANT+ FE-C and/or Bluetooth Smart to enable apps like Zwift, Rouvy, and The Sufferfest to control the resistance for structured workouts, virtual routes, and e-racing.

Simulated shifting is a feature smart bikes have that smart trainers do not. Using buttons on handlebar-mounted "brake hoods," you can shift gears the way you would on your outdoor bike. This technology is steadily evolving, including the ability to program your gearing and customize the buttons to replicate Shimano, SRAM, or Campagnolo shifters. As apps and indoor smart bikes continue to evolve, simulated steering controls and incline/decline are likely to become more mainstream.

Adjustability

Indoor smart bikes were developed with high performance in mind, which is illustrated by the attention paid to adjustability. With an indoor smart bike, you have the opportunity to micro-adjust handlebar and saddle positions, including the tilt of the bars. More importantly, you can use your favorite drop bar, flat bar, or aero bar instead of the stock setup. This not only allows you to replicate your outdoor position more accurately, but also means you can experiment with new positions and equipment to see if they are comfortable and powerful. You can do this outdoors, too, but it's far more convenient to do it indoors where you have your tools and spare parts, and you can leave your outdoor setup unchanged as a control. Some indoor smart bikes also have adjustable crank length so you can match the cranks you ride outdoors.

THE GOLDEN RULE FOR INDOOR CYCLING EQUIPMENT

As you can see, there are a lot of great options when it comes to indoor cycling equipment. Before going down the rabbit hole of researching the minute details of different models of trainers, smart bikes, and interactive apps, there is one Golden Rule for deciding whether a piece of equipment, a class, or an app is right for you: **The best indoor cycling options for you are those that increase the number of days you ride or increase the total amount of time you spend riding.**

If the social component of in-person studio classes is what excites you, a coach-led class that prepares you for the demands of your goal events will be a better investment of your time and money than the most high-tech indoor smart bike. If your personal and professional schedule means in-person classes and outdoor group rides are out of the question, a smart trainer or smart bike paired with an interactive app can allow you to participate in virtual group rides and competitive e-races instead of training in complete isolation. And if alone time is what you crave in this ever busier and interconnected world, you can still strip indoor cycling down to just you and the trainer. The range of options has never been greater, and once you find the equipment that works best for you, it's time to set up your indoor cycling space and plan your training.

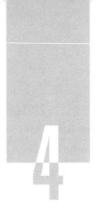

SETTING UP YOUR SPACE

Indoor training spaces are often as unique as the people who use them. Some athletes have elaborate "pain caves" with widescreen TVs, high-powered fans, and racing mementos hanging on the walls for inspiration. Then there are riders who carved out a little space in the garage or living room, with enough space to perch a laptop nearby. Some indoor cycling studios feature sound and lighting systems to rival dance clubs, and other venues are converted warehouses. You can improve your fitness and performance in any of these environments, provided you set it up correctly. How you arrange your space makes a big difference in the effectiveness of your workouts, and more importantly, how frequently and consistently you will get on the bike.

MAKING YOUR SETUP WORK FOR YOU

The best case scenario for riding indoors is to have a dedicated space where you can leave the trainer and associated equipment set up between rides. While there are some very motivated athletes who don't let inconveniences deter them from completing their workout, having to drag the trainer, fans, bike, and more out from storage before every ride is too high a barrier for many. This process gets even more labor intensive if you have to protect the floor or carpet from sweat or you need to reconfigure all the app-to-trainer-to-device connections each time.

When looking around your home for a space that will work, be sure it meets these absolute minimum requirements:

- **Floor space.** Floor space should measure at least 4 feet by 8 feet, which is only slightly larger than a twin bed.

- **At least one electrical outlet.** At minimum you need the ability to plug in a fan. If you are using a television, laptop, multiple fans, and a smart trainer, you'll need a power strip or multiple outlets.

Technically, your bathroom or closet could meet these conditions, but that doesn't mean they are good choices. Although you don't need a lot of floorspace to create an effective indoor cycling setup, a larger or more open space is preferable for airflow.

AIRFLOW

Keeping cool is the number one priority for effective indoor cycling workouts. Heat production during exercise can be 15 times higher than the heat your body is producing right now at rest, but your core temperature can only increase by 3–4°F before the stress of hyperthermia diminishes power output and your brain dials down your motivation to continue.

The sidebar on thermoregulation describes how the body responds to heat. Two of the primary ways the body cools itself are through the evaporation of sweat and the gradient between skin and air temperature, both of which are heavily dependent on airflow. When you are riding outdoors, you have plenty of air flowing over your body as you move forward, but sometimes even that is not enough. For instance, riding in a headwind increases airflow over the body relative to your speed. On a hot day that is good because it increases cooling, but a headwind on a cold day can be unpleasantly frigid. The opposite is true with a tailwind. On a hot day a tailwind reduces airflow over your body, so while you may enjoy going faster, you also risk overheating. Riding indoors in relatively still air is the worst-case scenario.

What about riding in a cold environment with no fans, like an unheated garage in winter? It's better than riding in a warm house with no fans, but you are dependent on the gradient between the temperature of your skin and the air around you. Initially, that gradient is big enough that you can dissipate a lot of heat. Pretty soon, however, you warm up a small pocket of air immediately surrounding your body and dissipate body heat more slowly. However, one benefit of training in a colder environment is that you can stay cool with fewer fans because moving cold air over your body dissipates heat faster than moving hot air over your body.

During strenuous exercise in a warm environment, an athlete can lose 1.5 liters of fluid per hour through sweating and respiration. Even if your sweat rate is far lower than that, there is likely to be some sweat on the floor when you are done with your indoor cycling workout. A bigger puddle of sweat is not a badge of honor; most times it means you did a poor job of creating enough airflow to facilitate evaporative cooling. Sweat that drips off your body carries with it far less heat than that same volume of fluid when it evaporates off your skin.

Increase Airflow with More Fans

A fan is a good start, but to maximize evaporative cooling two or three are even better. There are three areas you really want to hit: head/face, front of body, and back. If you have one fan, aim for as much coverage as possible over your head and the front of your body. If you have two fans, aim one at your head and the other at your body. And if that's not enough or you have access to a third fan, the most overlooked area for airflow is your back.

No matter how many fans you have, it is important to prioritize cooling your head and face. Thermal stress is a major limiter for athletic performance. In a 2011 study, 40 km time trial performance was nearly two minutes slower, and mean power output decreased by 6 percent when ambient temperature was 32°C

Heat is the enemy of performance, meaning that keeping the body from overheating is one of the best ways to improve athletic performance. Thermoregulation is one of the most researched aspects of sports science, particularly because strenuous exercise produces a lot of heat. Skeletal muscles are not very efficient when it comes to producing mechanical work. Even the best cyclists can only achieve a mechanical efficiency of about 20–25 percent on the bike. So, after all of your efforts, 75 percent of the energy you produce is lost as heat. The body has to get rid of heat rapidly in order to keep your body temperature, which is normally 97–99°F (36–37°C), from rising more than a few degrees. It is not uncommon for core temperature to exceed 100 degrees during strenuous exercise in a hot environment, but once you reach about 102 degrees, the thermal stress will diminish power output and the motivation to continue.

Understanding thermoregulation will help you see why the design of your indoor cycling setup matters. There are four primary ways you can move heat away from your body to the environment: evaporation, convection, conduction, and radiation. To start with, blood moves heat from core body tissues to the skin, and during exercise, vasodilation dramatically increases blood flow to the skin for more rapid heat exchange. Some heat is emitted as infrared radiation. Evaporation of sweat off your skin carries heat away as energy is required to vaporize water. Conduction happens when there is a temperature gradient between your skin and something touching your skin, like a wet cloth. If the cloth is cooler than your skin, heat moves down the gradient to the cloth. Convection works with a temperature gradient as well, but from your skin to air moving around you.

As your immediate environment gets hotter, the temperature gradient between your skin and the environment gets smaller, which means radiation, conduction, and convection become less effective. Evaporative cooling, which is always important and happening even when you're not visibly sweating, becomes even more important when ambient temperatures are high.

When you are setting up your indoor cycling space, you want to maximize the opportunities to dissipate heat through all four methods. Sweating alone can't keep up with the heat production. That's why a relatively open space with lots of airflow from fans is important, and why I don't recommend indoor cycling in rooms purposely heated to near or above normal body temperature unless an athlete is following a prescribed heat acclimation protocol.

compared to 17°C (90°F and 63°F, respectively), but it is not just a physical problem. The perception of thermal strain is enough to reduce time to exhaustion and reduce power output, potentially because it increases perceived exertion and reduces motivation. Some studies that have tested the perception of thermal strain applied menthol to athletes' faces during time trial efforts. Even when neither skin temperature nor core temperature was affected, time trial pace or time to exhaustion improved. The menthol is thought to stimulate cold receptors in the skin to induce a cool feeling, which reduces the perception of effort and allows the athlete to continue working at a high intensity.

I am not suggesting indoor cyclists need to start rubbing menthol on their faces to get a good workout. The point is, a fan pointed at your face and head not only aids in evaporative cooling, but the sensation of your face feeling cooler plays a role in perceived effort and motivation to continue riding.

Move Away from Heat Sources or Turn the Heater Off

Depending on the time of year, air flowing from nearby HVAC vents could be good or bad. In the winter, you may find it unpleasant to have hot air pumping into a room where you are trying to stay cool. If it bothers you, consider closing heater vents or turning the heat off while you're on the bike. In the summer, those same vents can be helpful if you also have central air conditioning.

SWEAT PROTECTION

As I mentioned when talking about airflow, it is likely sweat will accumulate on your bike and the floor during indoor cycling workouts. If you are setting up a training space in a room with carpet, it is a good idea to put a waterproof mat under the bike. When training in a room with a hard floor (concrete, hardwood, laminate, tile), you can still use a waterproof mat if you'd like, but an absorbent towel/rag will also work and reduce cleaning time. Just don't leave a wet towel or puddle of sweat on a hardwood floor.

The floor isn't the only thing you have to protect from sweat, nor is it the most important. Salty sweat is corrosive to all the metal parts on your bicycle or indoor cycle, to varying extents. Aluminum will oxidize, and steel will rust. Metal frames are typically protected by paint or coatings, but sweat can reach the metal through scratches and gouges. Carbon fiber and titanium frames and parts are relatively immune to sweat corrosion, but the steel and aluminum parts and fasteners are not. Brake and derailleur cables and housing, as well as cable ferrules, are susceptible to corrosion. Though the carbon fiber in your frame is corrosion resistant, carbon fiber in contact with alloy and salt-water can cause galvanic corrosion of the metal. Wiping sweat off your bike or using an absorbent "sweat net" that catches sweat before it drips onto your frame minimizes much of this corrosion. Don't forget the headset; sweat can seep in and degrade lubricant and damage the metal components of cartridge bearings. And an often-overlooked area is the bottom bracket; a lot of sweat ends up there due to gravity.

The binder bolts in your stem, seat post, and water bottle cages are a big concern when it comes to sweat corrosion. When these bolts corrode, they can seize in place, which makes adjustment or disassembly for travel difficult. When sweat gets between your frame and seat post, the seat post may seize into the frame and be very difficult to move. Corrosion will eventually weaken these bolts, which is particularly dangerous for the bolts that hold your stem in place.

The biggest potential risk is that sweat will corrode your aluminum handlebar. Although the bars are anodized to protect them from sweat, scratches or imperfections can allow corrosion to start. Handlebar tape prevents some sweat from reaching the aluminum, but sweat also gets trapped between the tape and bar. Because the bar is hidden under the tape, the damage can go unseen for a long time, sometimes long enough that the handlebar eventually breaks. Damage to that extent is rare, but is more of a risk for bicycles that are used exclusively for indoor training. Replacing your handlebar tape once or twice a year is a good idea anyway, and provides an opportunity to inspect your handlebars for corrosion.

NOISE

If you really want to make yourself unpopular in an apartment building, ride a trainer or rollers on a bare floor with the television volume cranked and two or three fans running. Oh, and ride at either 4:30 a.m. or 9:00 p.m.

Indoor cycling can be very noisy, but there are ways to make it quieter and less irritating to your family or neighbors.

- **The trainer itself.** Smart trainers and indoor cycles that have electro-magnetic resistance can be the quietest options available, although there will still be noise from your drivetrain (direct drive models) or your rear tire against the resistance roller. Wind and fluid trainers are louder.

- **Location.** There's also the issue of vibration, which can make any option louder if there is open space below the floor you're training on, like your downstairs neighbor's apartment. A basement or garage floor will cut down on noise from vibration. If you're training upstairs, invest in a thick mat to put under the trainer to absorb some of the vibration.

- **Entertainment.** Wireless headphones are one of the best things to happen to indoor cycling. Not only do they block out some of droning noise for you, but they also relieve everyone in a two-block radius from having to listen to your playlist or old Tour de France videos.

CONNECTIVITY

To use a smart trainer or apps while you are riding inside, you're going to need electricity and an internet connection. The apps that connect to the trainer use Bluetooth Smart and/or ANT+, so if you're just using the trainer and the companion app, you don't need an internet connection. To stream content or communication through an app (like Zwift) or to a device (like Peloton), an internet connection is required. Similarly, if you want your training data to sync to an app after your workout (like Strava or TrainingPeaks), you'll need a data connection via cellular data or internet access.

Keep in mind, depending on the devices and apps you are using, there may be restrictions on the number of Bluetooth connections that can be supported simultaneously. Different combinations of trainers, sensors, and apps have unique setup methods, but thankfully once you have your setup dialed in, the connection process should be quick.

You may need to consider a device to extend the range of your household Wi-Fi. Many people set up their indoor cycling space in a basement, garage, or extra bedroom, which can be far from the Wi-Fi router. A strong internet connection is beneficial, particularly for streamed content and interactive trainer experiences like Zwift and Peloton. If a web-based app is controlling your smart trainer and the connection drops, it can be very disruptive to your workout.

KEEPING EXTRAS WITHIN REACH

When you ride outside on the road or trail, stopping and putting a foot down is pretty normal. Yet, some cyclists and triathletes have a perception that riding inside has to be nonstop. It doesn't. There's nothing wrong with hopping off the bike for a minute to fill a water bottle, use the bathroom, stretch, or just take some time off the saddle. However, if you are participating in a virtual group ride or indoor cycling class or competing in an e-race, you might not want to get off the bike at all. When selecting and setting up your trainer space, it is helpful to have a counter or table within reach.

Speaking of arranging your stuff, the location of the device you watch—television, laptop screen, smartphone—can make a big difference in terms of comfort and performance. The ideal scenario is that your cycling position indoors is the same as your cycling position outdoors. (As mentioned in Chapter 3, whether you are using the same bicycle for both or have a dedicated indoor setup in addition to your outdoor bike, measurements like saddle height, handlebar height, and reach should be the same.) What many cyclists overlook, however, is how the position of the screen or screens they are watching affect the riding position. When you are outside, you are looking forward and keeping your neck in a position that's comfortable enough to maintain. What we see when riders move indoors is that screens positioned for watching television and movies are too high for a cyclist to see in their normal cycling position. You end up sitting up higher and craning your neck to watch the screen, which is not only uncomfortable but changes your biomechanics on the bike.

To position your data and entertainment screens, start by riding the bike in your training space using as natural a cycling position as possible—like you're outside. Then put your screens at the height that corresponds with your normal field of vision in your outdoor cycling position. Just as you keep your eyes on the road or trail, perhaps the screen will sit a little lower than handlebar height so your line of vision is similarly angled.

HEAT ACCLIMATION

An indoor cycling space can be an important component of a heat acclimation protocol if it is cold where you live and you are preparing for a competition in a hot or humid place. Before going any further, however, it is important to have some perspective. In terms of priority and impact on performance, remember that fitness, rest, nutrition, and hydration all come well before heat acclimation. It works, but it's time-consuming, an added complication, and—when done incorrectly—can do more harm than good. So, what I tell athletes is to focus first on being stronger, well rested, well fed, and well hydrated. If you've done all of that and still have time, then you can consider heat acclimation.

Acclimatization is a passive process that happens when you live or move to a hot environment. Acclimation, on the other hand, is an active process where you are creating conditions meant to stimulate the body's normal response to living and exercising in heat. If you live in Alaska and you are training for a summer event in Texas, acclimating is the only way to achieve some of the heat-related physiological adaptations before your event.

Prolonged exposure to heat, whether passively or proactively, stimulates a number of physiological changes that allow you to ramp up your mechanisms for dissipating heat. Some of them include:

- **Increased plasma volume.** Blood plasma is your body's reservoir for sweat, and more plasma means more fluid to carry heat from muscles and organs to the skin more quickly.

- **Earlier onset of sweating.** Sweat production starts sooner and ramps up faster to keep body temperature from rising too rapidly in a hot environment.

- **Increased sweat rate and perfusion.** You sweat more, faster, from more places.

- **Altered sweat composition.** Sweat glands adapt to pump out more fluid but retain some electrolytes. You still lose sodium through sweat, but not as rapidly.

- **Improved comfort.** Exposure to heat modifies perception of thermal strain.

To achieve these adaptations, or at least attempt to, athletes preparing for hot weather competitions spend time passively sitting in saunas as well as time exercising in heated rooms. One way to do that is through indoor cycling in a dry sauna, a bathroom, or a shower area. A typical protocol would call for an athlete to gradually increase time spent in a heated environment to 90–120 minutes a day over 7–14 consecutive days. Incorporating aerobic exercise into some of those exposures increases the benefit. If you remain living in a cool environment, the positive effects of acclimation only last about a week before diminishing rapidly over the next two weeks. However, the benefits of acclimation can be mostly retained by heat exposures every few days after the initial period.

If you are considering implementing a heat acclimation protocol in your training, I recommend working with a knowledgeable and experienced coach. The timing relative to your event date and the way you integrate it into your performance training make a big difference. The risks are not insignificant: training quality can diminish during the protocol, recovery can be hindered, hydration status is harder to maintain, and it adds physical and mental stress. So I will repeat what I tell all athletes: focus first on being stronger, well rested, well fed, and well hydrated. If you've done all of that and still have time, then you can consider heat acclimation.

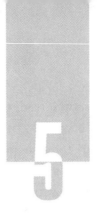

FOUR WAYS TO RIDE INSIDE

The best equipment in the world won't help you get faster and more fit unless you use it. Missing workouts is, by far, the biggest reason athletes fail to reach their goals. Maybe your training programs could have been better structured or you could have eaten differently, but there is no way to make up for training you never did. Coaches don't always admit this, but if they're being honest they will acknowledge that in their first season working with a new amateur athlete, getting that person to miss fewer sessions and sleep more are bigger factors for improving performance than any specific block of workouts. It's not that the workouts aren't important, but rather that consistency leads to stronger training stimuli and an overall increase in hours spent training, both of which will improve performance even if an athlete is doing the "wrong" workouts.

Consistency and compliance are such crucial metrics that if push comes to shove, I prioritize an athlete's ability to complete training ahead of creating the optimal training schedule. The great thing about training is that there are usually several routes to reach the same destination. If you have less time to train, we can adjust the intensity to create greater workload in less time. If you can only train Friday through Monday and have to take Tuesday through Thursday off, we can work with that. Riding inside is often a good way to increase training consistency because your indoor setup is ready to go whenever you are, unaffected by the weather outside, the hours of daylight, or the cycling club's ride schedule.

How you choose to ride inside can also impact training compliance. In the Dark Ages, indoor cycling meant being totally isolated, cooped up in your basement or garage slaving away to the droning noise of your rollers or old-school resistance trainer. If you were lucky, you had an old television and VCR or DVD player so you could watch movies or tapes of old races, or follow along with an indoor cycling video workout. Indoor training was a test of commitment, and indoor hours provided a measure of a rider's badassery.

The isolation of indoor cycling created stark differences in springtime fitness. Riders who trained more consistently by riding indoors showed up to spring races with more training hours and higher fitness than those who couldn't muster the motivation to spend hours spinning their legs in the basement. As the equipment and technology for indoor cycling have improved, the process of riding indoors has become more appealing.

To be successful in sports, you have to love the process, not just the outcome. You spend more than 90 percent of your time training for events that take up less than 10 percent of the annual hours devoted to your sport. So, if you are going to spend considerable time training indoors, you can't just approach it from the Dark Ages "embrace the suck" attitude.

If the only reason you ride inside is because you are forced to by the weather or your schedule, every ride will be a test of your determination. That's exhausting, and over time it is unsustainable. Your equipment and environment determine the types of indoor cycling you can complete, but finding appealing ways to ride inside is critical for long-term consistency.

You can divide the ways you can ride inside into four categories: off-grid, connected, interactive, and together. Each has its pros, cons, and best-use scenario, and you can sometimes ride in multiple ways using the same equipment. Some athletes may prefer or be limited to one category, whereas others may be able to utilize them all. As you determine your training goals and options for indoor cycling equipment, here are ways to take these four categories into consideration.

RIDING OFF-GRID

Technology has made a world of information available at our fingertips and enabled people to connect in real time from just about anywhere on the planet. You can shop 24 hours a day and have products delivered to your home in less than a day. You can answer emails from the backcountry. You can watch almost any movie or TV show ever made, on demand. The news comes at you at an unrelenting speed. It is no wonder a growing number of people are seeking ways to unplug, even for a little while. Endurance sports provide opportunities to create literal and figurative distance between you and the stresses and connections of daily life. Rolling out of the driveway or away from the trailhead is the way many people take some time to be unreachable and unplugged.

The current popularity of indoor cycling is the result of technology, including smart trainers, virtual routes with realistic graphics, and livestreamed group classes. But just because indoor cycling can be a high-tech endeavor, that doesn't mean it needs to be. There are even instances where riding inside off the grid is the best option for your training.

I think of riding inside off the grid as doing a workout without a connection to the outside world. It can mean riding old-school equipment, like rollers or a fluid resistance trainer, or using a smart trainer that's connected to a cycling computer or phone app but not streaming content. Riders should still record training data with a heart rate monitor and bike-mounted power meter connected to a cycling computer or through a smart trainer. That way the data can be uploaded to your favorite training software once you're done.

PROS

Sometimes you might be riding off-grid out of necessity. Not everyone has access to electricity where they are training or has a smart trainer and internet-enabled apps. When you want to use a resistance trainer or rollers in a parking lot for your prerace warmup, you most likely won't be using a smart trainer (unless it's one of the few self-powered models) or streaming training content to your phone. Other times, you might choose to ride off-grid for the following reasons.

There's Nothing to Stop You

The time and hassle of connecting all your indoor cycling hardware and software can be a barrier to getting on the bike at all. It might sound silly, but I can't tell you the number of times I've asked a cyclist or triathlete about a missed or shortened workout and been told they blew 15–20 minutes troubleshooting connectivity issues. Their internet connection dropped. The Bluetooth on their phone couldn't find the trainer because it was connected to a wireless speaker. They had trouble downloading a workout video. Their kid logged them out of the Apple TV, and they couldn't remember their password.

Now, most people iron out their connectivity problems and develop a routine for consistently and quickly getting their devices ready to go. Nevertheless, fewer things to connect means fewer opportunities for glitches that slow you down.

It's All Up to You

I've mentioned this before, but you have to call upon internal motivation to hit intensity targets when riding an old-school trainer or a smart trainer that is either in level/resistance mode or controlled manually from a companion app or cycling computer. In this case, it's not just that the trainer isn't being controlled in erg mode, but that you don't have anyone to compete or keep up with, there's no group training atmosphere, and there's no one there to encourage or push you. You are alone. That can be a challenge for athletes who rely heavily on external cues for motivation. It can also be an advantage for athletes who are easily distracted in group settings.

Training completely alone and with minimal entertainment (no music or TV/video) helps to prepare endurance athletes for the tough times during competitions when you have to turn inward to find the will to continue. It helps you get in touch with the thoughts and mantras that work for you, as well as the negative thoughts you will likely have during competition. Distractions make you reliant on the distraction instead of teaching you to channel your inner monologue to leverage positive thoughts and redirect negative ones.

CONS

The hard part about riding off-grid is that you are completely dependent on willpower. For some athletes, some of the time, that's no problem. But in 40 years of coaching I have yet to meet an athlete who has never succumbed to his or her negative thoughts. Willpower fails eventually, and that point of failure can be shortened by fatigue, hunger, overheating, and lifestyle stresses.

Skipping an interval set, easing up before the end of individual intervals, or just skimming 10 percent off the top of your target power outputs might seem like a minor transgression. In the grand scheme of things, I guess I would rather an athlete take these shortcuts than skip a workout altogether. However, if you are shooting for an ambitious training goal and if you have limited training time, these transgressions can add up over a period of days and weeks and effectively stall your progress.

BEST-USE SCENARIO FOR RIDING OFF-GRID

Short, high-intensity workouts focused on sprints (10–30 seconds), accelerations (10–60 seconds), or VO_2max intervals (1–4 minutes) are good choices for riding off-grid because these are maximum-intensity intervals that are best executed by perceived exertion. A smart trainer in erg mode isn't as useful for a sprint workout because you want to sprint as hard as possible, not at a specific target power. These workouts are also very engaging, even without outside entertainment or direction, because it takes focus to keep track of the timing of short intervals. It may be easy to zone out or lose focus during a 20-minute lactate threshold interval, but you have to pay attention when the workout is a series of 30-second intervals separated by 15 seconds of recovery.

RIDING CONNECTED

The next step along the technological continuum is riding inside while streaming content to a smart trainer or connected indoor cycle. In this case, I am referring to consuming training content rather than interacting with other users in real time. An example of riding inside connected would be completing a structured workout with the Zwift, TrainerRoad, or The Sufferfest app controlling your smart trainer. This is the primary way cyclists and triathletes execute structured workouts on a smart trainer or connected smart bike.

PROS

The greatest benefit from riding connected but by yourself is the increased engagement from streaming training content. Whether it is the graphics from a virtual route, video footage from a race or famous mountain climb, or the ups and downs of the interval workout bar graph that holds your attention, it's worth it if it means you'll stay on the bike longer or execute a higher-quality interval session.

When you ride connected, your workout data is automatically recorded and synced to the cloud. To facilitate this process, you can also connect your devices and apps to centralized fitness trackers, like TrainingPeaks and Strava. Having all your training data together in one place is critical for accurately monitoring training stress and tracking progress. Although it may seem surprising, one of the biggest problems coaches have with cyclists, triathletes, and runners who train outdoors is getting them to upload the data from their devices. Your data does you no good sitting in the device. And if you ride outdoors and indoors, or across multiple disciplines, but only upload some of the information, the holes in your data will make it hard to create an accurate picture of how you are actually doing.

Not only can you follow an individual structured workout when riding inside connected to an indoor cycling app, but you can also follow an entire training plan. Whether you create or select a training plan that features structured workouts or have a coach build you a personalized plan, some apps—including Zwift and RGT Cycling—will sync with your structured plan so you can ride each workout in the correct sequence.

CONS

Being connected to streaming content can be more engaging than riding off-grid, but the accountability and motivation components are still largely left to your willpower, particularly if you are using the level or resistance mode for a structured workout or free riding along to a video or virtual course. If you are using a smart trainer in erg mode to follow a structured workout, the trainer will keep you at your target power outputs, and you won't have to rely on willpower to complete the intervals correctly.

The other potential issue with riding inside connected is that it requires a reliable data connection so you can stream the content. If a web-based app is controlling the trainer and the connection drops, or the Bluetooth or ANT+ connection from your trainer drops, the app thinks you stopped pedaling. This leads to gaps in your training files, although that isn't too big of a problem. The bigger potential problem is that a trainer in erg mode will either stay at the target power from the moment the connection was lost or release erg mode altogether. You could end up in a hard interval that never ends or have your interval end prematurely.

BEST-USE SCENARIO FOR RIDING CONNECTED

This is a great way for an athlete to remove the need to remember a workout. Instead, you just select your workout and start riding. If you have longer intervals at a specific target power, like 10-minute efforts at 300 watts, you can turn on erg mode and settle in to your preferred cadence. If you prefer to use a power range, like doing those same 10-minute efforts at 300–315 watts, switch to level mode.

Riding inside connected is also the best method for preriding a simulation of a real course you will later experience in competition. These simulated courses—either accompanied by video or graphics—give you the opportunity to test out different pacing strategies.

RIDING INTERACTIVELY

Whether you are riding inside off-grid or connected, you are still going it alone. It's just you and the machine—even if the resistance is being controlled by an app. Adding an interactive component to riding inside has been the real game changer. Community, social connections, competition, and a sense of belonging are all part of the appeal of participating in sports. For a long time, riding inside meant severing those connections and being isolated in your basement, garage, or guest room. Isolation is not fun, which is why we turn to entertainment from movies, training videos, and apps with virtual routes.

Athletes don't take big steps forward in training because of epic individual workouts or competitions. They make progress by showing up day after day and accumulating month after month of solid training. Sometimes you will feel powerful and fast, your workouts will be fun, and your motivation will be high. Other times your training is going to be hard, and you're going to be tired and stressed. No matter how important your goal is to you, there will be days when you would rather stay on the couch than get on the bike.

PROS

Having a training partner is beneficial whether you feel great or feel like quitting. With the development of web-enabled cycling apps and smart trainers, indoor cyclists can finally communicate and interact with other riders, despite being physically alone. If you have the equipment to ride inside interactively, here are the reasons you should do it.

You'll Show Up More Often

It's easy to skip a workout when the only person you're letting down is you. When there is someone waiting for you at your favorite coffee shop or the group ride is gathering on the corner, you show up because they are expecting you. Training partners are great for creating accountability and giving athletes the nudge needed to get on the bike and out the door. That accountability works in a virtual environment too.

Virtual group rides via web-enabled apps give you something to commit to, and more importantly, a group of riders you can commit to. The beauty of virtual group rides is that they can be scheduled any time. The typical real-world group rides start in the morning after sunup, like your Saturday morning club ride, or later in the evening after work, like your local "Tuesday Night World Championships." It's hard to arrange a real-world group ride before work on a weekday, but you can connect with them to do a predawn virtual group ride.

Scheduled e-races on Zwift and live indoor cycling classes, like those available through Peloton, are also effective for making people commit to getting on the bike at a specific time, particularly if your friends, training partners, or teammates are going to show up too. Both incorporate two-way communication so riders can communicate with a class instructor or other riders in the class or race.

You'll Push Yourself Harder

There's a reason competitive cyclists and triathletes record their best power numbers during competitions and group training sessions. Even though the conditions when you are training on your own could be more conducive to setting PRs, athletes are able to dig deeper and sustain hard efforts longer when there are other riders to match or beat.

And it's not just the desire to win or be the best that makes riders push harder in a race or group exercise environment. In 1926, psychologist Otto Köhler discovered that weaker members of a group would try harder to match the performance of the group's stronger members, which led to improved performance in tasks that required contributions from everyone. The motivation gain to prove you're not the weakest in the group became known as the Köhler Effect, and as endurance athletes, we see it in action all the time. In the middle of the pack, no one wants to be the weak link that lets a gap open up in the paceline. At the back, no one wants to get dropped.

The Köhler Effect is one of the reasons group workouts are so important for cyclists, runners, triathletes, and swimmers. And if you are looking to improve your own performance, you don't want to be the strongest person in the group. A study by Irwin et al. compared cycling performances when riders were cycling alone and then with a virtual "partner" who they were led to believe had ridden 40 percent longer in the solo ride. The subjects had managed to ride an average of 10 minutes in the solo trial, but rode 9 minutes longer when they were motivated to keep up with a virtual partner perceived to be stronger.

The aforementioned study is in line with a larger body of research that shows that weaker members of a group improve their performance most when the group is working on a collaborative task where success depends on contributions from all members. Sounds a lot like a breakaway or a paceline, doesn't it? In a group that's not necessarily working collaboratively, like a generalized pack of cyclists, a virtual group ride, or a livestreamed indoor cycling class, the Köhler Effect still results in a motivation and performance gain for weaker members of the group—whether they are actually weaker or just perceive themselves to be weaker.

Interactive indoor cycling experiences provide multiple opportunities for creating motivation. You can catch, pass, or try to keep up with other riders' avatars. You can compete in e-races or compete against your previous performances on designated segments and virtual climbs. For the data junkies, you can track all your data right on the screen in real time and see where you rank on live leaderboards.

Just like in real life, sandbagging by riding in a group that's too easy for you might make you look good and stoke your ego, but it won't help you get faster. To get faster, you have to ride with and against riders who are faster than you. Finding those faster riders can be a challenge depending on where you live and the size and depth of the local cycling or triathlon community. Interactive indoor cycling gives you access to riders from all over the world, which essentially guarantees you can find a group that can kick your butt.

You'll Stay Connected to Your Community

Being an athlete is an important part of your identity, and in many cases the cycling, running, or triathlon community is an athlete's primary social connection with other people who identify as athletes. Unless you work in the outdoor industry, it is likely your coworkers think you're crazy for riding 100 miles at one time, or even 50. There are a lot of people in your personal and professional lives who don't understand endurance competitions and ask every summer whether you're going to ride the Tour de France this year.

The people in the endurance sports community understand you, have similar passions, and speak the same language. While having one or a handful of training partners provides accountability and opportunities to increase motivation, being active in a larger community provides an overall sense of belonging and social support system.

Interactive indoor cycling apps can be very effective for social support and encouragement. You don't have to know the other people participating in an e-race or virtual group ride, or the other riders riding along a virtual route, in order to give or receive kudos in real time. Groups can leverage the community engagement by creating challenges and milestones that can be celebrated. In the Peloton community, for instance, people are encouraged to call attention to completing their 100th Peloton ride so others can celebrate their accomplishment. Other communities use badges and other methods that identify riders' accomplishments and display them so other members of the community can acknowledge them.

CONS

The only real downside of riding inside interactively is that, just like doing too many outdoor group rides or even too many races, doing too many virtual group rides, free rides on virtual courses, or e-races can leave too little time and energy for focused training. You will maintain or even increase generalized fitness, but you will miss out on the benefits of accumulating time-at-intensity from structured interval training. Triathletes and time trialists must be especially wary of high-intensity, competitive group rides. They can be counterproductive to your goals. Interactive indoor rides are great to integrate into a training program on occasion, especially for the training fun and variety they provide, but they are not great as the basis for a training program.

From a technical standpoint, you face similar potential drawbacks as riding inside connected. You need a reliable data connection, there are subscription costs for the apps, there is time required for setup, and although you can free-ride and communicate with others on Zwift at any time, the specific times for e-races, virtual group rides, and streaming classes may not match up with your schedule.

BEST-USE SCENARIO FOR RIDING INTERACTIVELY

E-racing, virtual group rides, and streaming group classes are the best uses for riding inside interactively, and they are really the driving force behind the increased popularity of indoor cycling. Smart trainers and app-controlled structured workouts were convenient and an improvement over old-school trainers, but the ability to interact with other cyclists without leaving your house was the game changer for indoor cycling.

RIDING TOGETHER AND IN PERSON

The fourth way you can ride inside is to physically go to an indoor cycling class in a performance center, a cycling studio, or your local gym. The experiences and workouts in these instructor-led classes can vary widely, from a dance party on pedals to a hard-for-hard's-sake sweatfest to a structured-interval set based on individual power zones. They all have their merits and target audiences, and they share some common benefits. Because riding together in real life, often with an instructor or group leader, involves more considerations surrounding your workout execution, we'll go a little deeper in our discussion.

LIVE LEADERSHIP AND COACHING

Having an instructor or coach at the front of the room provides opportunities for personalized encouragement, as well as direct accountability. If you are slacking off, a live instructor can step in and help you refocus. If you are doing well, having a coach or instructor look you in the eyes and call you by your name can be very effective for boosting your motivation and performance. Participating in an indoor cycling class can also be a good way to get instruction on cycling form, pacing, and how intervals work.

FINANCIAL COMMITMENT

You pay for what you value and value what you pay for. Making a reservation for an indoor cycling class creates a financial incentive to actually show up. This is the same reason I encourage athletes to register for their goal events early. Once skipping a workout or an event is going to cost you money, you are more likely to find a way to get there.

While there are membership or per-class costs associated with indoor cycling classes, they can be a great option for athletes who don't have the room for an indoor setup at home, can't afford the upfront cost for their own equipment, or who aren't going to be riding indoors frequently enough to justify buying their own equipment.

FIXED SCHEDULE

When you are training on your own, you can ride indoors anytime. Even when you are streaming workout content, you have a lot of flexibility. There are virtual group rides and e-races that start throughout the day and night. On-demand indoor cycling classes can be streamed at any time. But the 6:00 a.m. indoor cycling class led by your favorite instructor, Kate, only happens at 6:00 a.m., so you have to get out of bed and go or you will miss it. The certainty of a fixed class schedule can be helpful because it becomes one of the things on your schedule that cannot be moved. The problem with being able to train at any time is that anytime can quickly become no time.

CAMARADERIE

People build meaningful relationships through shared experiences and often attribute greater value to an experience done with others even if no relationships are built in the process. One of the frequent gripes that event promoters hear is, "I could ride these roads any day of the week, why should I pay you so much to ride them during your event?" That's true, you could. You can run a marathon anytime you want to, and in many cases, you can run on the course used for competition. You can complete a 140.6-mile triathlon on your own as well. But those accomplishments are more memorable and fulfilling when there is a real finish line and other athletes, friends, and fans to cheer you on.

Group training environments are supportive and uplifting. The workout is often very difficult, and having a person next to you doesn't make it any easier, but the difficulty is more acceptable because you are not doing it alone. If the person next to you can stick it out, you can too. And afterward you have this shared experience to talk about and compare notes.

HOW TO CHOOSE AN INDOOR CYCLING CLASS

Once you have decided to participate in indoor cycling classes, you have to find the right class for you. If it is just one class here or there, or while you are traveling, then you don't really need to be picky. There's no harm in occasionally jumping into a class that is just a dance party on pedals if that's what you are looking for or if the alternative is not being active at all. If you want to integrate indoor cycling classes into your training program in a way that adds to your performance, then evaluate them based on the principles of training: stress/recovery, specificity, individuality, and progression.

Stress/Recovery

Throughout your entire training plan, your progress depends on applying training stress and then allowing for adequate recovery. This works at the granular level of intervals and recovery periods up to the arrangement of training and rest days in a week, and finally to your monthly and annual plan. Indoor cycling workouts at gyms and fitness studios, and those available on demand, can be well structured in terms of work-to-recovery ratios or they can be hard for the sake of being hard. When the primary goals are to make people sweat and finish the class with the sense they worked hard and burned a lot of calories, then you'll find the work-to-recovery ratio skewed to more work and less recovery. But instead of creating a more effective training stimulus, efforts that are too hard, too long, or too frequent—with insufficient recovery between them—just reduce your actual power output. Perceived exertion may scream zone 5, but with insufficient recovery, you will soon be producing zone 2 or zone 3 power outputs.

Check in with the instructor: What you are looking for is an instructor who can provide a clear rationale for a workout structure, other than it's going to make you sweat and be really intense. Even better, if you are looking to attend a cycling class on a regular basis, find out if the classes follow a plan or if there is a schedule that lists the workouts for each class.

Specificity

Athletes who are looking to improve performance for cycling events need to attend indoor cycling classes designed to meet the power demands of the events they are training for. For competitive cyclists and triathletes, this often means looking for a performance center or cycling class run by a coach. These classes may not be as entertaining because effective interval sets are often not the most fun, crowd-pleasing kind. The intensities will be consistent and repetitive instead of all over the map, and while you may do some pedaling out of the saddle, no sport-specific class will have you doing pushups on the handlebars. For the greatest specificity, you should either be using your own bike on a trainer or have the opportunity to adjust the indoor cycle to be as close as possible to your normal bike fit.

Ask about how training data is gathered. Do you need or can you use a bike-mounted computer to record your own training data? Are you logging into a system at the facility that will control the trainer or record training data and give you access to it afterward? Can you use your own pedals, or do you need shoes with cleats that match the equipment at the facility?

Individuality

The principle of individuality simply means your training has to be personalized to your physiology and your personal needs. While the process of applying training stress and allowing time for recovery and adaptation works for everyone, there is tremendous variability in how individual athletes respond. Training history, current fitness level, genetics, fatigue, and where you are in relation to a goal event all play roles in what workouts you should be doing and how you respond to training stress. Training is not one-size-fits-all, but indoor cycling classes sometimes are, at least in terms of when they are scheduled and the workout everyone does together. This can present some challenges, but there are ways you can make a group class more individualized.

Look for a power-based class where your target power outputs are established by a performance test (typically the first class) or entered manually, and are customizable if necessary. That way, if the workout features three 10-minute zone 4 intervals, everyone in the class is riding the intervals based on his or her individual functional threshold power (FTP). Whether you reach the target power outputs on your own or are in erg mode depends on the technology being used for the class. Classes can also be run by heart rate or perceived exertion.

A good coach or instructor will keep a close eye on riders in a group class and adjust the workout for individuals when necessary. In the example of the 3 × 10-minute zone 4 interval workout above, a coach may have less-experienced riders drop to a recovery pace after 8 minutes instead of 10 or make other adjustments on a person-by-person basis.

The ideal class atmosphere is also highly individual. Some athletes thrive in an aggressive environment where they are being implored to push harder and give more. Others prefer minimal guidance from the instructor but like being able to focus on the music. Some are looking to feed on the enthusiasm from the instructor and their classmates. When the environment and atmosphere are right for you, you will look forward to going to class, you'll feel safe, supported, and encouraged during class, and when it is over, you will be glad you went—even if you are exhausted. Any class environment that is cruel, belittling, or resorts to shaming as a means of motivation should be avoided at all costs (and shut down so no one else is harmed).

Progression

Progression goes hand in hand with stress and recovery, in that the amount of training stress required to stimulate a positive adaptation increases as your fitness improves. As you get stronger, you have to manipulate the intensity and duration of intervals and workouts in order to generate enough workload to continue making progress. Indoor cycling classes marketed as a 4-, 8-, or 12-week training plan are going to feature progression, and the workouts will take into account the returning participants' developing fitness. In health clubs or cycling studios where there are a lot of classes, but attendance is intermittent, the focus is more on stand-alone classes, and the programming tends to be more static. Many clubs have a mixture of both: classes that are singular sweatfests and seasonal or theme-based classes that follow a training plan.

WHAT'S THE BEST WAY TO RIDE INSIDE?

The best way to ride inside is the way that entices you to ride more often and be more consistent with your training. All four types can play a role in developing the fitness and power required for optimal performance, but they are just tools, apps, and methods. The next step is learning to structure training, determine your intensity zones, and create a plan you can follow.

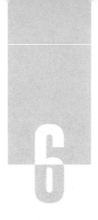

FIT AND FAST,
INDOORS AND OUT

Now that you've learned about fitness fundamentals and the equipment, bikes, and apps you can use to enjoy your training inside, let's drill down a bit deeper by getting into three more details that must be understood to train purposefully and effectively both indoors and out: the basic concepts of training, the measurement of workout intensity, and how stress can help you become more fit and fast. By the time you're done with this chapter you'll be ready to move on to Chapter 7, where you can design your workouts or know enough about workout planning that you can purchase a premade plan that is right for you.

TRAINING BASICS

On the surface, deciding what to do for a workout is pretty easy, regardless of whether you're indoors or outside. Whether you're an Olympian or brand new to cycling, there are only two questions to ask yourself: How long will I ride, and how intensely? From those two decisions your workout is almost ready to go. Of course, as you know, there are a few other things to determine, such as the ride's purpose, whether it's a steady ride or one with intervals, if it's on hills or flat roads . . . and more. We'll get to all of these details later. For now, let's just deal with the basics of the ride—duration and intensity—and a few other related matters.

DURATION

This is an easy part of planning: How long will the ride be? The most common way of answering this is deciding how much time you'll be in the saddle for today's ride. You may want the ride to be long or short—or somewhere in between. Of course, "long" and "short" are very individualized. For a rider who does ultra-endurance rides, a short ride may be 3 hours long. But if you're a recreational rider, "short" may be 20 minutes. The same goes for long workouts.

If you're new to cycling, let's say within your first three years of riding, duration is the most important part of the ride. By gradually increasing the duration of your long rides, your fitness will improve—as long as you are consistent. If you miss a bunch of workouts, regardless of the reason, you'll likely have to take a step back and begin increasing your long-ride durations again. That's because whenever you miss a workout, your body loses a little bit of fitness. If you miss several, there will probably be a significant loss of endurance. The body has a way of returning to previous levels of fitness whenever it can. But if you ignore the loss of fitness resulting from several weeks (or perhaps only a few days) of missed rides, you'll likely suffer when trying to pick up where you left off. It's better to start back conservatively by making the next long ride a bit shorter than what it would have been had you not missed the workouts.

INTENSITY

There's a bit more complexity to workout intensity than there is to duration. And just as with duration, we need to measure it in some way. Of course, clocks are much easier to use than the heart rate monitors and power meters that measure intensity. Let's first look at a simple and commonly used method of measuring intensity: identifying how hard the workout *feels* to you. You might ask, is this really a way of measuring a workout? Yes, it is. And it's been around for a long time.

In the 1950s a Swedish psychology professor at Stockholm University, Dr. Gunnar Borg, had an idea for a way people could express how hard any effort feels. Its first application was in the medical field, but athletes and coaches soon adopted it as a valuable tool for measuring intensity. It's still widely used

FIGURE 6.1. Borg's 0–10 Rating of Perceived Exertion (RPE) Scale

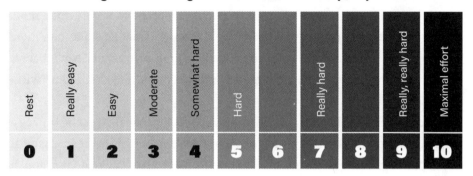

Rest	Really easy	Easy	Moderate	Somewhat hard	Hard		Really hard		Really, really hard	Maximal effort
0	1	2	3	4	5	6	7	8	9	10

in endurance sports today. Borg's tool is called the rating of perceived exertion (RPE) scale. Whenever athletes work out, they can label the effort they are experiencing with a simple number.

Early in his process, Borg developed a scale ranging from 6 to 20 so that the ratings could relate to heart rate: He would multiply the rating by 10 to estimate the person's heart rate at that time. For example, an RPE of 14 would predict a heart rate of 140. That didn't always prove to be true. Later, he came up with a scale of 0 to 10. This is more popular with athletes today and a bit easier to use, and it doesn't involve heart rate. It's only a simple scale of how you feel while exercising. Figure 6.1 illustrates Borg's 0–10 scale.

Let's give Dr. Borg's RPE descriptions a bit more context by looking a little closer at his intensity levels of 3, 5, 7, and 9. At an RPE of 3 the effort is "moderate." That means you could probably maintain this intensity level for a long time, perhaps for a few hours. At 5 the exertion is "hard." You could probably do this for a fairly long time, maybe a couple of hours of steady riding or somewhat more when highly fit. Most riders could ride steadily at an RPE of 7—"really hard"—for perhaps 20 to 40 minutes. A few very fit riders could hang on for up to an hour, but they'd be really hurting near the end. An RPE of 9 is "really, really hard." The typical duration for this intensity is about 1 to 5 minutes, depending on how fit the rider is.

You may recall from Chapter 2 that there are three ways of expressing an endurance rider's fitness: aerobic capacity, anaerobic threshold, and economy.

Your aerobic capacity is about 9 on Borg's 0–10 scale (you could probably sprint for a few seconds when you reach your aerobic capacity, so it isn't quite a 10). Anaerobic threshold occurs around 7—"really hard." Now let's add one more term to give more meaning to training intensity: aerobic threshold. Note that it's *aerobic* and not *anaerobic*. The first means "with oxygen," and the second "without oxygen."

The aerobic threshold occurs at an RPE of 3 to 4 on the 0–10 scale. During a gradually increasing intensity, such as during a warm-up, this is the intensity at which you first notice that your breathing is a bit elevated. You're no longer just taking it easy. If we align all three of these physiological markers with Borg's 0–10 scale, we get Figure 6.2.

Another simple way of measuring intensity that is commonly used by some riders is the talk test. If you're riding with a partner and you can't talk, you're probably above your anaerobic threshold. That's an 8, 9, or 10 RPE. If riding alone (you probably don't want to do this with anyone nearby!), sing out loud the song phrase, "happy birthday to you." If you can barely sing all the tune's six syllables before taking a breath, then you are probably close to your aerobic threshold—a 3 or 4 on the RPE scale, or lower. If you can't get out all six syllables before sucking in some air then you're probably above your aerobic threshold—5 to 7 RPE. Not very scientific, but it works. Try it on a ride to get the hang of it.

FIGURE 6.2. **Physiological Effort Markers and Borg's 0–10 Scale**

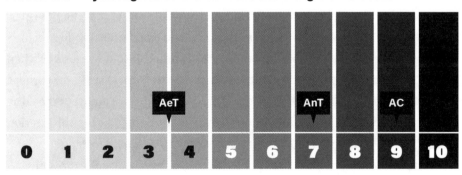

AeT: Aerobic threshold   **AnT:** Anaerobic threshold   **AC:** Aerobic capacity

FREQUENCY

Now we have the basics of a workout determined—duration and intensity. In every workout you'll ride for a certain amount of time and at a certain intensity. That's simple. Let's move beyond this and discuss what happens when we put several days of workouts together, as in a week of training. To do this we have to introduce the concept of frequency.

Frequency is nothing more than the number of times you work out in a period of time, such as a week, which is the most common time frame for this term. Some riders work out every day. That's a frequency of 7. Others take two days off every week to rest. Their frequency is 5.

VOLUME

Combining frequency with duration is called *volume.* When you tally all of the workout durations you did for a week, you're measuring volume. World-class riders such as Tour de France competitors typically have a volume of more than 20 hours per week. Thirty is not unheard of for them. First-year novices may have a volume of 3 hours per week, or even less. Everyone else is in between these extremes. This, again, is a good marker for the new rider to keep track of over time and work to increase. But be careful of pushing yourself to the point that you no longer recover after a day or more of rest. That's a dangerous situation called overtraining, which we'll come back to later in this chapter.

TRAINING LOAD

Adding together your weekly volume and your total weekly intensity gives you your *training load.* That's a measure of how hard your training was when taking everything into consideration. The challenge in doing this is measuring intensity. When it comes to training load, RPE just doesn't quite hack it. That's when the more sophisticated intensity measuring tools such as heart rate monitors and power meters come into the picture. And that's where we are going next.

EFFORT, HEART RATE, AND POWER

Borg's RPE scale and the talk test do pretty well when all you are doing is telling a buddy how hard your ride was. But it's not very handy when trying to describe your training load for the week. And training load is key. As your training load increases, so does your fitness—as long as you don't overdo it and wind up overtrained. You'll recall that training load is the product of your weekly volume and your intensity. Volume is easy to measure. Not so for intensity. The two most common methods of precisely measuring intensity on the bike, and therefore knowing your training load, are heart rate and power. Whether you're riding indoors or out, or a combination of both, if you want to know your training load and therefore how your fitness is progressing, then you need to use one or both of these tools when riding. While both are indicating the intensity of the ride, they really aren't telling you exactly the same thing. Let's see why.

HEART RATE

The first heart rate monitor that could be worn during a workout was invented in 1977 by a professor at the University of Oulu in Finland. Dr. Seppo Juhani Säynäjäkangas's new device was intended for the Finnish cross-country ski team. But it caught on worldwide. By the mid-1980s the Polar heart rate monitor was being used by athletes in a wide range of sports, including cycling. The heart rate monitor is still the most popular intensity-measuring tool for endurance athletes everywhere.

Heart rate measurement is quite individualized, as everyone's heart doesn't beat at the same rate under the same conditions. You can be riding side by side on the road with a training partner, but your heart rates could be significantly different. In order to make heart rate measurement meaningful across the board, an individualized reference point is needed. There are two common ways of establishing that reference point. One way is to find your maximum heart rate. The other is to determine your anaerobic threshold heart rate. From this, and using percentages of that reference number, you set up training "zones"—small ranges of heart rate that coincide with Borg's 0–10 RPE scale.

Which of the two reference points is better? I'd argue that your anaerobic threshold is much more telling than max heart rate, and it's a lot easier and safer to find. Why? Let's look at an example. Two athletes may have the same max heart rates but considerably different anaerobic threshold heart rates, which is pretty common. If their zones were set up the same way and based on max heart rate, and they did a workout in zone 4 (a certain effort level that typically includes anaerobic threshold), one athlete could easily be at 6 RPE on the scale while the other is at 8. One rider's workout is "hard" while the other's is "very hard." Zones based on one's anaerobic threshold heart rate solve that problem.

But now you have a new task—to determine your anaerobic threshold heart rate. The old way of doing that was to have a test done on a cycling ergometer using sophisticated equipment in a laboratory, as described in Chapter 2. It would certainly work, but there are obvious downsides: practicality and cost. Being tested in a lab is not cheap. But there's a simpler—and cheaper—way.

Sports scientists have known for decades that a rider can stay at his or her anaerobic threshold for a long time, perhaps for an hour. Some highly fit riders can hang on for as long as 75 minutes, and less fit athletes for perhaps 30 to 40 minutes. In the early 2000s, Andrew Coggan, a sports scientist and cyclist, used this roughly one-hour concept to come up with a simple way to determine anaerobic threshold. If the athlete does a time trial race that takes about one hour, the average heart rate for that race would be a good indicator of anaerobic threshold. And there's no cost, other than the entry fee. But what if there was no race scheduled? Couldn't the rider simply go as hard as possible for one hour? In theory, yes. But in actuality, probably not. The missing ingredient is motivation. Races are highly motivating. Solo rides aren't. Experience tells us that a rider doing a one-hour, nonrace, solo ride at max effort will actually go about 5 percent easier than he or she would in a race. The motivation to push one's limits just isn't there. That's why Coggan came up with an alternative test that can be done as a workout. It requires that the rider go as hard as he or she can for 20 minutes and then subtract 5 percent from the average heart rate. (This test is described in the appendix's "Field Test Main Set" section.)

Because Coggan's 20-minute test is not done by measuring oxygen levels, it's not an anaerobic threshold test. Nor is it a lactate threshold test as described in Chapter 2 because no blood samples are drawn and tested. So he called it the "functional" threshold. Today his functional threshold idea has caught on, and we have intensity measurements throughout the endurance sports world such as "functional threshold heart rate" (FTHR), "functional threshold power" (FTPo), "functional threshold pace" (FTPa) for running and swimming, and "functional threshold speed" (FTS).

Once you've tested and know your FTHR you can set up training zones as described in Chapter 8. Your FTHR can also be used to determine your training load. We'll come back to that a little later in this chapter.

Interestingly, once your FTHR is known, we can roughly estimate your *aerobic* threshold heart rate by subtracting 30 beats per minute from your FTHR. For example, if your FTHR is 150 beats per minute, your aerobic threshold heart rate is around 120. This is just a rough estimate, but it's close enough for our purposes. This comes in handy when doing aerobic threshold workouts as described in the appendix in the "Aerobic Endurance Main Sets" section.

If you've been using a heart rate monitor for some time, you are probably aware that heart rate responds slowly to increases in intensity. It lags behind rapid changes in speed or power. It's not very sensitive. For instance, when you sprint, you might've already finished the sprint before your heart rate shows you how hard it was. But for steadily paced rides a heart rate monitor is nearly perfect. At any given moment you know how hard you are working by glancing at it. Intervals that last five minutes, for example, can be monitored using heart rate. But if the interval is only 30 seconds long, heart rate is of little use.

We should clarify some other aspects of heart rate training, too. Let's start with the idea that a low heart rate is good. When riding indoors at any given speed or power, if your heart rate is lower than it was in previous workouts under the same conditions and at that same speed or power, then you are more aerobically fit. This means that as you get in better aerobic condition it becomes harder to get your heart rate up into a high training zone. Unfortunately, athletes often think this means they have poor fitness since they can't get their heart rates up. It's just the opposite. But if you sincerely want to get your heart rate to rise more easily in training, lose fitness by taking a week off from riding (I'm not recommending that you do this, as I don't really want you to lose fitness). Your heart rate after that break will be higher at any given speed or power and will rise quickly with changes in intensity. We know this probably seems counterintuitive, but that's how heart rate works in training.

POWER

The bicycle-mounted power meter was invented in 1987 by Ulrich Schoberer, a German mechanical engineer and cyclist. It took about 20 years for it to catch on in cycling sports, and now it's widely used by riders. It's also found on some indoor training machines. You may have one on your road or mountain bike. Power meters are used with zones much in the same way a heart rate monitor is used. Once your functional threshold power (FTP) is established, your training zones can be determined (see "Field Test Main Set" in the appendix for details). This is where using heart rate and power begin to differ a bit.

Over the course of the season an experienced rider's heart rate zones will change very little, if at all, even though fitness may change considerably. Zone 3 at the start of the year will be much the same as zone 3 at the end of the season. Power zones, however, change quite a bit with changes in fitness. While you may notice that the two sets of zones overlap early in the year, they are likely to separate as your training and fitness advance. Improving fitness means increased power output, but not increased heart rate or RPE. When at your AnT (see Figure 6.2), your heart rate will be the same as it was earlier in the season and it will still feel "really hard," but if your fitness has increased, your power output will be greater.

Let's take a deeper look at power zones. Recall from Chapter 2 that the biomechanics of pedaling indoors with a wind-resistance, magnetic, or fluid trainer that has no flywheel are not the same as when riding outdoors. We explained that when riding such indoor machines, the rear wheel immediately slows a bit every time your pedals come to the 12 and 6 o'clock positions. So you have to push just a little harder at the start of the downstroke to get the wheel going again. On the road this is not necessary due to the momentum of the rear wheel. An indoor trainer with a flywheel accomplishes about the same thing as riding outdoors because the flywheel maintains some of the wheel's momentum. Without a flywheel on your indoor training machine, your economy—the energy cost of pedaling the bike—decreases as compared with riding outdoors on the road. That means one of the three markers of fitness is compromised. It's sort of like saying that you are "less fit" when riding such indoor trainers, even if you really aren't. If you seem to be less fit when riding indoors, then your power training zones shouldn't be set at the same levels as when outdoors. All of this is just to say that you may need two sets of training zones: one for indoors and another for outdoors. It's also likely to be the case if you have different power meters on your indoor machine and a bike used only on the road. It's likely they won't agree. I know that's a hassle, but it's necessary for meaningful training. If you just use your road zones when riding indoors, the workouts are likely to feel much harder than on the road, and you'll soon find you are dreading indoor rides. That leads to missed or shortened workouts and decreased fitness. It's important that you have both outdoor and indoor training zones. This, of course, means testing both outdoors and indoors. I'll get into that in Chapters 8 and 9.

STRESS AND FITNESS

What does being "more fit" mean? Let's look at it this way: A workout is stressful. If you're more fit, then you can manage more stress. This is obvious when you do a hard ride. Your RPE, heart rate, and power are high, so you feel the stress. In contrast, easy workouts are low stress. There's still some stress, but not nearly as much as when riding fast at a high effort. Following a stressful workout, if you allow for some rest and recovery—especially sleep—your body adapts to the stress by growing stronger. Your fitness increases.

GOOD STRESS AND BAD STRESS

If your aerobic fitness is increasing, as determined by comparing workout power and heart rate for similar workouts, then training, whether indoors or out, is going as it should. When this happens, what you experience is a gradual increase in fatigue over time. That's good stress, or in the language of sports science, "eustress." It's also called "overreaching," meaning pushing just a bit beyond your physiological limits. After a couple of weeks of this good stress, you need an extended break from training—some rest and recovery lasting a few days. This will clear away the fatigue, and you'll be ready to get after it again in order to create more fitness.

Then there's bad stress. You're probably familiar with the word "overtraining." It's not the same as overreaching. Overtraining is a more extreme level of stress than overreaching. When overtraining, you are pushing well beyond your physiological limits. This is likely to happen when you decide to skip a rest-and-recovery break and keep on training hard. This is "distress," meaning "bad stress." When overreaching, your accumulated fatigue will go away with a few days of reduced training load. But when overtrained, the fatigue won't go away. You're lethargic and tired all the time. It's like you are sick. The symptoms can last for weeks. There's no way you can train. In fact, just getting out of bed in the morning can be difficult. Overtraining is not to be taken lightly. The bottom line is that you shouldn't skip recovery days or planned breaks from training of a few days.

THE TRAINING STRESS SCORE

To avoid overtraining, athletes need to monitor their training load to prevent the excessive and prolonged stress caused by overly hard workouts combined with inadequate rest-and-recovery time. So, how can you know how much stress you are experiencing? After all, you can do a very short-duration workout that is very high in intensity, or you could go for a very long-duration ride at a low intensity. Then there are all of the rides between these two extremes. How do you gauge the stress your body is experiencing on a daily and weekly basis? Is it good stress or bad stress? The duration part of the equation is easy to measure, but intensity is a bit more difficult. And both are necessary to know how stressful your workout was.

Measuring workout intensity brings us back to heart rate and power. Knowing one of these tells you how intense the workout was. These tools are much more precise than using RPE, although it's still important to always be aware of your perceived exertion while riding. But when it comes to knowing exactly how intense a ride was, your average heart rate and average power provide excellent data. Knowing average heart rate or power for the workout, however, is only meaningful when you compare it with your personal reference point—your functional threshold heart rate or functional threshold power. There are rather lengthy formulas for all of this, which we won't go into here. This calculation of workout intensity can be done automatically on most cycling-focused training websites if you upload your heart rate monitor or power meter data to them. With your ride data, they can tell you what your exact intensity was for the ride.

This brings us to something called the training stress score (TSS). This is a tool used by almost all online apps intended for indoor or outdoor riding. These apps can tell you precisely how hard you are training. Since every workout is stressful to some extent, all we need to do is calculate that stress by measuring the two components of every workout discussed earlier—duration and intensity. Duration is easy to measure. How many hours, minutes, and seconds did the ride last? And as you know by now, intensity is a bit more difficult to measure. Using TSS makes this easy, and the app does the calculating for you.

You can total the daily training stress scores for the week and know what your training load is. In fact, the app will do this for you, too. And be warned: TSS values are highly individualized. What is right for you may be too much or too little for another rider. Once you determine a safe level of weekly total TSS, you can make small increases, such as 10 percent, each week for two or three weeks before taking a rest-and-recovery break for three to five consecutive days. Then start the next training block at a slightly higher training load than you started the previous training block. This will ensure that you are overreaching and not overtraining—developing some eustress, not distress.

You should now have a better understanding of the big picture of training. You are ready to start looking more closely at the specifics of your rides. After all, being knowledgeable is the starting place for better self-coaching. So now let's get down to the details of where the rubber meets the road (or the flooring, if you are indoors): building your training with purpose.

PURPOSEFUL TRAINING, INDOORS AND OUT

This chapter is all about having a purpose to your training. That may be something you've given little or no thought to—before now. Through years of experience in training cyclists, it's become obvious to me that those who know what they want achieve more than those who don't. Why do you ride a bike? Why do you spend a significant amount of your valuable time sitting on a saddle turning cranks? It's probably because you see a benefit, such as excellent health, endurance for long events, faster riding, or a place on a race podium. I'll show you how your goal can be realized.

So, first, have a goal. You've undoubtedly heard this many times in your life. There's a good reason for that. Goals point you in the right direction and can help keep you focused. You've probably heard this too: A goal has two parts—what you want to achieve and when you want to achieve it. You may have tried setting goals before and not achieved them. I'm going to show you how to create and follow a plan that will get you to your goal.

That you are reading this book tells me that you are probably looking for some direction to help you grow as a rider. The starting place for this chapter is knowing what you want to accomplish and when you hope to see it achieved. That's entirely your call. I can't be of much help there, but I can show you how to plan for the goal's achievement. Let's get started with your plan.

FITNESS AND HIGH-PERFORMANCE PREPARATION

Let's start by taking a 30,000-foot view of your season, or the macro cycle of your training plan. From well overhead we'll try to get a view of where you want to go with your training. All of this starts with your goal. If you are a competitive rider, you probably have an event that you're aiming for. You want to do well on that day. If you ride for fitness, your goal is probably along the lines of achieving the highest levels of performance, endurance, and vigor possible. And more than likely, you'll know when you are there by how you feel throughout the day—including, perhaps, how easy it becomes to climb that tough local hill or even the six flights of stairs to get to your office. In either case you will benefit from having a training plan designed in such a way as to foster improvement. This training plan will contain periods of more and less effort and saddle time throughout the season or year. I'll also show you how to use different types of workouts so that they aren't the same old, same old, day after day.

THE TRAINING PLAN

High performance in cycling, as in almost everything in life, is most likely achieved when following a plan. It is seldom the result of random training by just getting on your bike a few times each week. Wishing and hoping just won't get it done.

If you follow discussions on online forums related to training, you've likely come across someone's comments about how the best riders and athletes actually don't follow a plan. The truth is, they do. A plan doesn't have to be on paper—or your computer—to be a plan. The best riders who have been training for years have a plan, but it's just stored in their heads. It's not some meaningless hodgepodge of random rides. Regardless of what these advanced riders may say about their disdain for thinking ahead, they know what they need to do and when they need to do it to achieve their goal in a timely manner. That's really what a plan is all about—preparing for the future. What most of these supposedly nonplanners are really good at doing is deciding how to modify their mental blueprints to better fit their current situations. But for some reason, age-group athletes and fitness riders often think of a seasonal plan as a rigid document that must be blindly followed regardless of the circumstances at any given time. Actually, it's not that way at all.

Seasonal planning should be thought of more as a highly flexible route to a known, or, more excitingly, a desired destination or end point. It's as if you are planning a long, cross-country drive to visit relatives in a faraway city. You could pull out and mark up a map to decide which roads and highways to take to get to your destination. Or perhaps, since you've taken this drive many times before, you don't need a map. You know how to get there. In either case, along the way, you are likely to run up against roads closed due to construction, new highways that just opened, heavy snow, flooding, or other impassable situations. When that happens, you will probably decide to take an alternative route. It's doubtful you would ignore the road closures and press ahead regardless. That's obvious.

As you go through your season or cycle following a plan, whether it's in your head or on paper or digitized, you must be ready to take a detour when something goes wrong. That something could be illness, injury, slow progress, rapid progress, unrelenting fatigue, family or career interruptions, or any number of other situations. When such disruptions occur in your training, you treat it just as you would any plan interruption, regardless of if or how the plan is documented. To do otherwise would be as foolish as driving on a closed road.

PLANNING INDOOR RIDES

A good place to start with your plan has to do with identifying which rides you will do inside rather than on the road or trail. These choices may be seasonal as the weather and daylight changes or done year-round. They can probably be decided now but be sure to adjust them as your needs change throughout the year.

The first step is to look at key workouts that you currently find difficult to include in your normal weekly routine, regardless of the time of year or weather, such as rides that require you to travel somewhere, either by car or bike, to find, for example, suitable terrain, streets uninterrupted by traffic or stoplights, or safe road conditions. These workouts are commonly intervals, steady tempo rides, and active recovery sessions. There could be other rides to move indoors, such as steady endurance-building rides that are hard to do where you live due to frequent stoplights or heavy traffic. Or the reason to go inside may be to do group rides when there are no such opportunities where you live. As you read about in Chapter 5, such group rides may now be done indoors with the right app and digital equipment. Let's now take a look at how to prepare a quick and easy training plan.

YOUR TRAINING PLAN

Now it's time to show you how to create a simple personal training plan to help you achieve your goal based on progressive training throughout a year-long season. You'll divide your year into periods with each having an objective that, taken together, lead you to your seasonal or annual goal.

As noted above, your plan can be on paper, on your computer, or in your head. The newer you are to the sport, the more important it is to commit it to writing. That's simply because you're taking a long drive to someplace you haven't been to many times—or ever. But even if you have been there many times before, the process of writing it down helps you to think your way through it and consider all of the alternatives relative to your needs. Paper (or electronic) plans are quite commonly used by the very best endurance athletes and their coaches.

Each period described here has a purpose: to develop some aspects of the fitness markers discussed in Chapter 2—aerobic capacity, anaerobic threshold, and economy. Figure 7.1 illustrates the general cycle of a plan and lists each period's common workout types. When planning for an event, you can identify the different periods by counting the weeks backward on a calendar, starting with your event date. For example, the last week leading up to your event is the "Event" week. The 1 or 2 weeks prior to that make up the "Peak" period. Use 2 weeks if your event is very long—for you—and you have a very high level of fitness. Otherwise, your "Peak" period would be 1 week. The "Build" period lasts 8 or 9 weeks. Make it 9 weeks if you are over age 50 and take a rest-and-recovery (R&R) week every third week. If under age 50 this period lasts 8 weeks with a R&R week every fourth week. Make your Base period 12 weeks long with R&R weeks every third

FIGURE 7.1. **Common Training Periods**

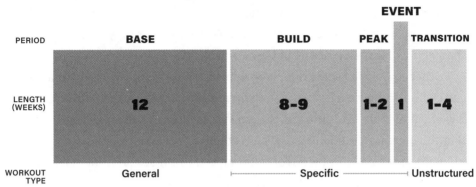

(over 50) or fourth (under 50) week. The details of these periods are explained in greater detail later in this chapter.

Refer to Figure 7.1 as we explore these periods of endurance training and the fitness-related goals of each. (For more details on planning, see my books *The Cyclist's Training Bible* and *The Triathlete's Training Bible*.)

Event Selection

As you can probably tell from the above discussion, planning is based largely on the event you are training for, such as a bike race, triathlon, gran fondo, or century ride. You may have a few of these planned for the months ahead. I recommend no more than about three such high goals in a season, though, because for each A-priority goal (usually a single, greatest priority in that season) you'll have to taper, meaning you'll shorten workout durations and reduce volume before such an event. A taper during a Peak period usually lasts 1 or 2 weeks. During this period you reduce the volume of your weekly riding. You'll shed fatigue so that you come to the day of the event on form, rested, and ready. Unfortunately, every time you taper, a bit of your fitness is lost. That's just the common physiological effect of reduced training, which can't be avoided when resting so you are fresh on the day of your event. This may seem contradictory to your event goal, but it's actually not a significant concern as fatigue is a much greater obstacle to high performance and can be lost quickly while fitness is lost at a slower rate with reduced training. Were you to taper more frequently than about three times in a season, you'd likely lose too much fitness. There may certainly be exceptions to the suggested three A events, but they are rare.

Other goals for a fitness rider may be increased strength on the bike, a weekend cycling trip with friends or family, or greater overall fitness. While you may have several goals. I recommend that you focus on one primary goal at a time so that you increase the likelihood of succeeding.

Before looking at the details of laying out a training season, I should point out that e-racing is changing things that athletes and coaches have taken for granted in endurance sports for decades. Traditional planning for a season has always been based on when outdoor races are scheduled. That was linked closely to the weather—spring classics in road cycling in northern Europe followed by grand tours in the summer, world championships in triathlon and cycling in late fall, and an "off-season" for both sports in the winter months. Indoor cycling severs the connection between seasons of the year and race season. It doesn't matter what the weather is when you are riding indoors. What I will describe in the following pages is the more traditional way to plan a season. If you are primarily an e-racing enthusiast, the concept described here still applies; you still need to develop fitness in a somewhat methodical progression. But the weather and traditional timing play no role in when the training periods occur.

With that caveat in mind, let's now dig a little deeper into the planning periods illustrated in Figure 7.1.

Base Period

The early season Base period typically lasts up to 12 weeks and starts 23 or 24 weeks before your A-priority event. This is your most important event (a stage race or multiday event counts as one A-priority event). The purpose of the Base period is to develop *general* fitness early in the season.

What is "general" training? It is made of workouts that are *unlike* the expected demands of the A-priority event or goal that you're training for. For example, if your A event or goal is short, punchy, and fast, such as a criterium or other short, high-intensity race, you would do long, steady, and slow rides throughout much of the Base period. The purpose then is to build aerobic fitness. In fact, even if your event is just the opposite—long, steady, and relatively slow—you should still do the long-steady-slow rides in the first 3 to 6 weeks of the Base period. In this situation, however, you should briefly venture into the shorter, higher-intensity intervals for the last few weeks of the Base period. The reason for doing the long-steady-slow rides early in Base is that it's important to have a good aerobic base, muscular strength, and pedaling skills before doing high-intensity or more specific training.

Of course, if you don't race or participate in events and instead have other kinds of goals as a fitness rider, you certainly don't have a need for tapering and being on form for competition. Your primary concern is pressing ahead with your riding to boost performance, endurance, and vigor. The Base period is excellent for this. Many fitness riders stay in the Base period doing general training for most if not all of the year. This produces great general fitness.

The appendix presents suggested workouts targeting six abilities—the key workout types that define race preparation. These are shown in Figure 7.2. The long, steady, and relatively slow rides may be found in the "Aerobic Endurance" category, while the high-intensity sessions are under the "Anaerobic Endurance," "Muscular Endurance," and "Sprint Power" categories. (All-out, out-of-the-saddle sprinting is not recommended for indoor workouts, but if you must perform them inside, I recommend that you do them on an indoor cycle rather than a bicycle on a trainer.) It's also common to do "Muscular Force" workouts in the Base period, especially in the first few weeks.

The other types of workouts to focus on in the Base period are in the "Speed Skills" category of workouts. As you'll see in the appendix, these are workouts intended to improve your pedaling skills, neuromuscular connections, and general coordination. Most of these are best done indoors. By the time you get to the next period—Build—you should have your skills quite well established for the season.

Build Period

The Build period typically lasts 8 to 9 weeks and is focused on *specific* event preparation—workouts that gradually become more like the demands of the A-priority event for which you are training. If you're doing a short, fast race, such as a criterium, your workouts should increasingly become very much like the race—short and fast. The best way to do this, besides the high-intensity intervals mentioned earlier, is to do other short, fast races. Only now these will be B- or C-priority races. For B races you should only reduce training in order to rest for about 3 to 5 days at most. For C races there is no rest break at all. They are treated like workouts. While you may want to limit how many B-priority events you do, there is little need to limit the number of C races in a season. They are quite good for your A-race preparation in the Build period.

For the athlete whose A event is long, steady, and relatively slow—such as a half- or full Ironman triathlon, or an ultra-endurance ride—the Build period is when such long, steady workouts become the focus of the training. High-intensity training, especially the anaerobic endurance sessions, should generally be done by athletes training for relatively short events that last less than about 4 hours.

During the Build period of the season, it is common for fitness riders to gradually shift toward doing high-intensity intervals. This typically does not need to last more than about 8 weeks as it becomes very difficult to make gains in such workouts beyond that number of weeks.

The fitness rider may also use the Build period to tailor training with workouts that gradually become more like the demands of the goal ride—perhaps a century, a weekend trip, or a fast group ride. If your anticipated goal ride has a lot of climbing, your workouts should increasingly involve heavier climbing and more wattage. The best way to do this is to complete other short climbs either virtually or on the road.

Following these weeks of higher-intensity training, the fitness rider may return to a Base period with an emphasis on aerobic endurance (AE), muscular force, and speed skills workouts to rebuild those abilities, especially AE, over about 4 to 6 weeks of riding. Then the fitness or recreational enthusiast returns once again to the higher-intensity training of the Build period. This alternation of Base and Build training can last for several weeks but should have a scheduled rest period in between to allow your body to adapt physiologically.

Peak Period

The Peak period is only used by the race-focused athlete, but it could be applicable to the fitness rider with a longer event, such as a century ride, gran fondo, or high-mileage gravel ride. During the Peak period, tapering to reduce accumulated fatigue is done for 1 to 2 weeks, and ride duration is gradually shortened so that by the end of the taper, the typical ride lasts only about half as long as was common in the Build period. This, of course, reduces the weekly volume of training. By reducing training duration—but not intensity—fatigue is gradually shed while event fitness is sustained at a fairly high level. I can't emphasize enough how important it is to keep your workout intensities the same as they were in the Build period. Intensity is now the key to keeping your fitness high.

Event Period

When you enter your event week, you're down to the last 6 or 7 days until your A-priority event. Now the purpose is to remove any lingering training fatigue while sharpening event readiness. The latter means an emphasis on intensity. Just as in the Peak period, the key to reducing fatigue is to shorten the duration of your workouts. In this period they are less than half as long as they were in the Build period. To come into form, your fitness intensity must remain high. That means doing workouts well below your anaerobic threshold (see Chapter 2) if you're preparing for a long, steady, low-intensity event, such as a full-distance triathlon or century ride. For very short, fast events, such as criteriums, these very brief workouts are now mostly done at about your aerobic capacity. For all other types of events, the workout intensities in the Event period are somewhere between Ironman and criterium intensities and should still be event-like.

Transition Period

Following your A-priority event, or perhaps your Build period for the fitness rider, it's time to take a break from highly focused and fatiguing training. The past few months of focused training have probably taken their toll on you not only physically but also mentally. You are likely to need some rest and recovery. This break from training may last just a few days or a few weeks, depending on where in the season you are—if you have more events on the schedule or if it's the end of the season. This may be a total break from training, in which you don't do any workouts. Or if that seems strange and you can't imagine not riding at all, you may do some short and very easy sessions. Once again, an indoor ride may be perfect for this.

THE ESSENTIALS OF PLANNING

You should now have a rather general understanding of how you're going to train in the coming weeks and months. This is based on your purpose for riding and when the general and specific workouts will be included in your plan. Understanding general and specific types of training is all well and good, but you need to be able to convert this knowledge to what you will actually do on the bike and when you'll do it.

This brings us to what I call the "basic" and "advanced" abilities in my *Training Bible* books. All of the workouts described in the appendix fall into one of these two categories, and they have a lot to do not only with your seasonal plan but also with your weekly workouts.

BASIC AND ADVANCED ABILITIES

My training approach envisions six fundamentals, or abilities, of endurance performance. When developed in tandem and with intention through training, you can expect to see growth in your athletic performance and reach your goals. Individual workouts are designed to target these abilities.

As shown in Figure 7.2, there are three basic abilities, located at the corners of the triangle: aerobic endurance (AE), speed skills (SS), and muscular force (MF). These three aspects of physical conditioning pertain to all athletic endeavors. They are the most essential, so working on them should generally precede any training done in the advanced category. The advanced abilities are on the sides of the triangle: muscular endurance (ME), anaerobic endurance (AnE), and sprint power (SP). These three advanced abilities are developed through high-intensity training. In most situations, you should work on them after working on the basic abilities in your periodization plan.

For most fitness riders, training in the basic abilities should make up the entire Base period, while the advanced abilities are limited to the Build period. For most competitive riders training for short and fast events, the basic abilities also take up the entire Base period. For other types of high-performance events, especially long and relatively slow ones, the basic abilities will only be done for a few weeks early in the Base period before high-intensity, advanced workouts

FIGURE 7.2. Basic and Advanced Abilities of Training

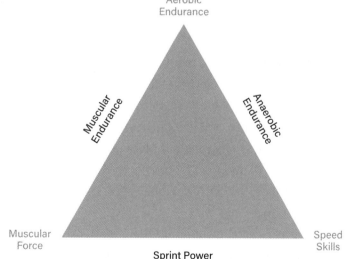

are included for the remaining weeks. Of course, since some events fall between these two extremes, there are many ways to arrange the abilities in planning. The underlying model for making this determination is that *in the Build period, your workouts should become increasingly like the event for which you are training.* As for the Base period, most, if not all, of the workouts are general and not necessarily like your event. Understanding and applying these guidelines is important for good planning and training. Again, for more in-depth guidance on this topic see my *Training Bible* books for cyclists and triathletes. I'll get a bit more specific on this topic of workout abilities and when to do them later in this chapter. For now, let's get a bit of a deeper understanding of the abilities.

ABILITIES AND FITNESS

Recall from Chapter 2 that there are only three physiological determiners of endurance fitness: aerobic capacity, anaerobic threshold, and economy. How do these compare with the six abilities? In other words, when you're doing a certain type of workout, which fitness marker is being developed? To start with, let's summarize the relationships in training to help you better understand the "why" of the workouts described in the appendix. As you read about each type of workout ability here, you may want to refer to the workout descriptions in the appendix to understand how a workout targets a particular ability.

Basic Ability: Aerobic Endurance (AE)

You may recall from Chapter 2 that there are two general ways to improve your aerobic capacity. You can do lots of long, relatively easy rides to improve your capacity for processing oxygen, and you can do short, very intense intervals. It's usually better if the low-intensity, long-duration rides precede the highly intense intervals. AE workouts fall into the first category—relatively low intensity with lots of hours in the saddle. See the "Anaerobic Endurance" ability section below for the interval workouts.

Long, easy rides can certainly be done indoors, but if you find that boredom is an issue, then these rides may best be done on the road. Of course, by now you may have changed your perception of indoor training as boring, having read about your many equipment and app options in Chapter 3. But if not fully convinced yet, the shorter, aerobic threshold sessions described in the appendix are great when done on an indoor cycle as there are no cars, stoplights, or dogs chasing you. There's nothing to interfere with your steady and focused training.

Basic Ability: Speed Skills (SS)

Speed skills (SS) are very closely related to the economy fitness marker as explained in Chapter 2. By improving your skills, especially your pedaling technique, you become more economical and waste less oxygen. Of course, even when you aren't doing SS workouts, you must remain focused on using good technique. It usually takes several weeks of concentration on a skill for it to become a habit. During that time, you must be focused on how you are pedaling. Once your pedaling skill is habitual, you won't have to concentrate on it nearly as much.

Not only are SS workouts recommended for indoor riding, but some of them, such as isolated-leg training, are generally best done indoors for safety.

Basic Ability: Muscular Force (MF)

Muscular force (MF) is the ability to drive the pedals down. The greater your muscular force production at any given cadence, the greater your power and the faster you ride. This is also related to economy: If you are able to forcefully drive the pedals down with no greater effort due to stronger muscles, you will be more efficient when it comes to oxygen usage. That's why speed skills and muscular force typically overlap in training, especially in the early Base period. MF training involves highly structured hill workouts and may also include strength training in the gym with an emphasis on combined hip-, knee-, and ankle-extension exercises such as squats, leg presses, and lunges. (This book won't get into the details of gym-based workouts, but you can find them in the *Training Bible* books.)

MF workouts may be done indoors, but you must have a trainer on which you can greatly increase the resistance on the rear wheel or, better yet, one that connects directly to your drivetrain. Of course, you can also do MF workouts on a smart trainer or indoor smart bike with the resistance set heavy. And indoor cycles with friction or magnetic resistance generally provide a stable platform for the heavy loads you'll be working under. On the road, these workouts involve overcoming the effects of gravity—going uphill—which, of course, isn't a possibility in the indoor environment.

Advanced Ability: Muscular Endurance (ME)

Muscular endurance (ME) is the ability to ride at or slightly below your anaerobic threshold for a relatively long duration. Notice in Figure 7.2 that muscular endurance is on the side of the triangle between the aerobic endurance and muscular force corners. There's a reason for this position. ME is to some extent the product of your AE and MF workouts. Once these two markers of fitness are well established, you are ready to do ME workouts. That's why basic ability workouts precede the advanced workouts. For performance riders who do steadily paced events that take approximately 45 minutes to 4 hours, such as triathlons and time trials, this is the most important ability of the Build period. For fitness riders and for those doing nonsteady events such as road racing, this is still an important aspect of preparation.

The typical ME workout involves a moderately hard effort done with long, steady rides—intervals of 5 to 20 minutes that, in total, tally up to about 40 minutes of combined intervals within a workout. By "moderately hard" we mean at a perceived exertion of 5 to 7 on a 0 to 10 scale. These are the types of workouts you'll find for ME in the appendix. Such workouts often require a significant amount of recovery—typically 48 hours or more—before doing another high-intensity session.

These are great sessions to do indoors since terrain, traffic, stoplights, and the many disturbances common on the road won't interfere with your concentration and completion of the workout.

Advanced Ability: Anaerobic Endurance (AnE)

As explained earlier, anaerobic endurance (AnE) workouts are the high-intensity intervals that also help to boost aerobic capacity. In fact, AnE workouts can bring your aerobic capacity to a peak. The work intervals may be as short as 30 seconds or as long as 4 minutes, with the recoveries between them of the same duration or slightly shorter. Typically, as these workouts progress, the recovery intervals get shorter. It's common for very fit athletes to only take recoveries that are half the duration of the work intervals as their training progresses. The combined work interval time may total 5 to 20 minutes within a single workout. Be very cautious with AnE workouts as they require a long recovery—at least 1 and maybe even 2 or more days of easy riding or days off for most riders. One such ride per week is often enough for many older riders. Of course, you may do an ME workout in the same week so long as there is adequate recovery time between them. AnE sessions also make for great indoor workouts. Please remember that to get the true benefit from these intervals you must be working in an anaerobic state; moderate-intensity intervals will not give you the same physiological benefit.

Advanced Ability: Sprint Power (SP)

As the name implies, sprint power (SP) workouts develop the raw power that make you fast for very short durations, such as a few seconds. This ability is very important in determining the outcomes of road races, criteriums, and some track events. Being positioned in Figure 7.2 between speed skills and muscular force tells you what is critical to SP development: economy. You must be able to turn the cranks at a high cadence (SS) with a great force (MF) being applied to the pedals whether in the saddle or standing.

Although you can do SP repeats while seated, doing them standing on an indoor trainer—wind-resistance, fluid, or magnetic—is not recommended for safety and economy reasons. The bike will not be able to move side to side as it does on the road, which means that you would be practicing something that isn't feasible outdoors and is therefore counterproductive economically.

Combined-Ability Workouts

A workout doesn't have to be focused on only one ability; there can be two or three in any session. One reason for this is that when you are riding in your A event, especially road races, all of the high-intensity abilities are likely to be challenged in back-to-back hard efforts. Such workouts prepare you for this. Second, if you are struggling to stay motivated riding indoors, changing up the abilities adds a lot of variety. A good example of this is combining three abilities into a single workout. The warm-up could easily morph into an aerobic threshold portion (see the appendix for details) followed by alternating SS and MF repeats. When working on advanced abilities, you can also combine workouts with a focus on a high-intensity portion (ME, AnE, SP) followed by a maintenance portion for one of the basic abilities (AE, SS, MF). I'll introduce this concept of ability maintenance a bit later in this chapter.

LIMITERS: WHAT'S HOLDING YOU BACK?

One of the fundamental training principles of sports science is "individualization." This simply means that athletes respond differently to training. You may do the same workouts as your training partner, but it's not likely that your bodies will respond in exactly the same ways. One of you may be more able to do very long aerobic endurance rides, while the other may be faster when it comes to anaerobic endurance workouts. Over time you'll simply respond individually to the workouts although they may be exactly the same. When it comes to training, our physiologies are unique in many ways.

It's obvious that we each have strengths and weaknesses as riders. These define who we are as athletes and, also, what we need to focus on (our weaknesses) in training to become more fit. When a weakness interferes with your goals, it is called a "limiter."

While there could be more variables involved here, such as lifestyle or nutrition, let's think of limiters in terms of the six abilities. If your sprint power ability is poor but sprinting is not important to your goals, such as when doing a triathlon, then it may be a weakness, but it is not a limiter. It's not holding you back

TABLE 7.1. What Is Your Limiter?

Ability	When the ability is a limiter, you . . .
Aerobic Endurance (AE)	Can't complete a "long" ride (relative to goal) or at least a 1-hour ride.
Speed Skills (SS)	Have poor pedaling skills or pedal in "squares" rather than "circles."
Muscular Force (MF)	Have difficulty with climbing short hills while seated on bike.
Muscular Endurance (ME)	Are unable to ride steadily at a moderate effort for more than 30 minutes (RPE 7; see Figure 6.2).
Anaerobic Endurance (AnE)	Can't ride at a high effort (RPE 9) for more than 2 minutes.
Sprint Power (SP)	Are unable to sprint competitively at an all-out effort (RPE 10) relative to other riders.

from achieving a training goal. If, however, you need to sprint faster in a road race to achieve your goal, then SP is a limiter and must be addressed in training.

You may have a pretty good idea of what your strengths and weaknesses are from reading about the six abilities in Figure 7.2 and thinking of how you perform on the bike. But just in case you don't, Table 7.1 may help you identify yours.

What you need to determine is which of these is a limiter. Everyone has a limiter, no matter how fit and fast they are. That ability must become the primary focus of your training. If it's an advanced ability, which is usually the case, the basic abilities on the two corners on either side of it in Figure 7.2 must be fully developed before concentrating your workouts on the limiter.

This doesn't mean you won't work on any other aspects of fitness. You will. They just won't get as much attention as your limiters. As you plan your training, this must always be uppermost in your mind.

MAINTENANCE WORKOUTS

It's important to explain one critical aspect of training briefly mentioned earlier—the maintenance of the abilities. This has to do with another sports science principle: reversibility. If you stop training an ability, the fitness gains made previously for that ability will gradually fade away. I suspect you are fully aware of this, but this leads us to a discussion of how the previously developed specific abilities are maintained throughout the season.

If you are in the Base period and your training is focused on AE, SS, and MF, you will be doing several of these workouts in a week. There could be two or three sessions of each. When you move into the Build period, your workouts may become more focused on ME, AnE, and SP. But now your predicament is that somehow you need to maintain the level of fitness of the basic abilities previously developed while concurrently building the advanced abilities. If you focus only on the advanced abilities, the basic ability fitness gains will erode. That's a dilemma. Let's see how it can be resolved.

Fortunately, the human body is a remarkable mechanism. If you do a certain type of workout often enough, it will adapt to the unique stresses of that workout. That's what makes us more fit. Changing your routine so you do the workout less frequently won't increase fitness, but it will maintain it. If you do a specific ability workout about half as frequently as it was done when you were trying to increase fitness, it will stay at a high level for a few weeks. This is only the case if that ability was brought to a high level of fitness before you started to reduce the related workouts. For example, if you do two long rides each week in the Base period and your aerobic endurance becomes well established, you can then do one such ride each week in the Build period and keep your AE at a high level. That's pretty cool. It means, however, that you can't forget the gains you made earlier in the season lest they go away later on. Every one of these maintenance workouts becomes critical to your progress. You need to keep this in mind as you get into planning your training, which we'll do shortly.

REST-AND-RECOVERY WEEKS

Continuous training without an extended break ultimately leads to the accumulation of fatigue. You become tired, and your training is less effective. Should the fatigue become great enough, you may become overtrained. As explained earlier, don't confuse overtraining with overreaching. The latter is necessary to become highly fit. The former actually results in a loss of fitness and must be avoided. Fatigue associated with overreaching goes away with a few days of rest. Overtraining lingers for weeks or months despite little or no training at all. It's like having a serious illness such as Lyme disease or mononucleosis. In fact, the symptoms of overtraining are quite similar to these diseases. That's nothing to be taken lightly.

How do you prevent this from happening? You build frequent rest-and-recovery (R&R) weeks into your training routine. These are a few consecutive days of greatly reduced training or even a day or more off from training altogether. I recommend that athletes do this every third or fourth week when following a focused training plan. Younger or experienced athletes can typically take a break from training every fourth week, while older or less experienced riders probably need R&R every third week. Which category do you fall into? Let's say that "younger" means under age 50 and "experienced" means three or more years in the sport. There are obviously going to be exceptions. If you're unsure, the only way to determine which works better for you—2 weeks or 3 weeks of training before an R&R break—is to experiment: Take the more conservative route at first—a training break every third week.

Most athletes need only 3 to 5 days of reduced training to rejuvenate the body and be ready to go again. How long your break lasts depends on how challenging your training was and how tired you were coming into it. This involves paying attention to how your body feels on a daily basis. This may be assisted by using any number of computer apps that daily measure such metrics as resting heart rate, heart rate variability, sleep status, and accumulated stress.

At the end of the R&R break you should feel well rested and ready to get back into focused training. But before doing so, I recommend you test your current fitness. The appendix provides common field tests that may be done to determine your status. These test results are used to reset your training zones as you head into the next 3- or 4-week block of training.

Whew! That was a lot of detail about the intricacies of effective training. Now it's time to finally lay out your plan for the season.

PLANNING FOR INDOOR AND OUTDOOR TRAINING

You should now be ready to start putting together your seasonal overview. Again, you can commit it to a paper or electronic version, or if you are highly experienced in such seasonal planning, it may require little more than a mentally stored outline. Next you need to decide what a common week of your training will be like in each period and lay out its plan on a daily basis. Once this is done for each of the periods, you are ready to start exercising with a purpose, or what we call training.

As previously discussed, certain workouts are better if done indoors since there are fewer variables, such as weather, traffic, and terrain, to contend with. Of course, what exactly those indoor rides may be about depends on your unique training environment and your plan. Some riders may need to do, or choose to do, nearly all of their training indoors, while others do most of it outdoors.

There are many ways to develop a training plan. Some are more complex and time intensive than others. I suggest a relatively easy way of planning your season based on weekly patterns by period. Then throughout each period you'll simply follow the appropriate pattern for 2 or 3 weeks before taking an R&R break from training. Remember to take the R&R break; this is not only where you rejuvenate but also where your body becomes stronger and adapts to the training load.

YOUR WORKOUTS

Before getting into the weekly patterns, let's consider three general categories of workout types that will help you determine how to design your weekly plans.

Limiter Workouts

As previously discussed, limiters are those abilities at which you are not quite as well developed as you need to be to achieve your fitness or performance goal. To refresh your memory, these are generally one or more of the advanced abilities for experienced riders. For those new to the sport, the basic abilities are likely to be limiters. Later in this chapter you'll see suggestions for doing a certain type of workout on certain days of the week, spaced fairly evenly throughout each week.

But given your limiter, you may decide to shift attention from an ability you are good at to your limiter so you get two or more limiter-related workouts in a given week. Keep this in mind as you study the suggested training weeks that follow.

Anchor Workouts

Anchor workouts are the ones you do every week on given days because of certain lifestyle restrictions. It could be that you do a group ride every Saturday morning, or perhaps you meet a group of friends on Tuesday evenings for an indoor cycling class. That's an anchor workout because it's the only day the group rides. Or there could be a day each week when you can't ride outside due to standing commitments and little available time, so you do a short ride indoors. That's also an anchor workout. You get the idea: An anchor workout is one that can't be changed.

Key Workouts

Key workouts are the most important rides of the week for you. They are the workouts you've decided are most important for you given your training goals and your limiters. They are most likely to be the advanced ability workouts. And since they are relatively high intensity, they need to be separated by one or more low-intensity days so that you recover adequately before going hard again. Of course, key workouts don't have to be high intensity. A really long ride at low intensity will certainly challenge you and require some recovery time afterward.

WEEKLY PLANS BY PERIOD

Now that all the planning details are covered, it's time to start considering how to arrange the workouts for the training weeks of each period in the season. I'll show you a typical week in each period for an experienced rider using the ability categories explained earlier. Of course, none of these may exactly fit your needs. We're all different in many ways from other athletes. There are empty weekly planning schedules in each period so you can begin to think your way through your personalized plan and pencil in your workouts. This may only require rearranging the workouts as suggested in examples for that period. With this in mind you should design your own unique weeks.

You may notice that earlier I identified five periods in a plan, but there are only four periods with suggested training patterns below: Base, Build, Peak, and Event (we also include Rest-and-Recovery weeks). That's because the fifth period, the transition, is intended to be unstructured, allowing you to remove the burden of highly focused training for some period of time following your season or cycle.

Note that the details of the various types of workouts listed here may be found under their ability headings in the appendix.

See the "Abilities and Fitness" section above for descriptions of each ability and what the abbreviations stand for in each of the following weekly training suggestions.

BASE

PERIOD LENGTH UP TO 12 WEEKS

Early Base Period Week
Event/athlete: Recreational and fitness riders; steady paced events, long- and short-course triathlon, time trials, centuries.

Mon.	Tues.	Wed.	Thurs.	Fri.	Sat.	Sun.
MF	SS	AE	SS	MF	SS	AE

Note: This is an example of a training week for the Base period for steadily paced events. This weekly training pattern should be used for the first 4 to 6 weeks of the Base period before switching over to the pattern shown below (late Base period week) for the remainder of the Base period.

Late Base Period Week

Event/athlete: Recreational and fitness riders; steady paced events, long- and short-course triathlon, time trials, centuries.

Mon.	Tues.	Wed.	Thurs.	Fri.	Sat.	Sun.
MF	SS	AnE	SS	MF	SS	AE

Base Period Week

Event/athlete: Variably paced events such as road races and criteriums.

Mon.	Tues.	Wed.	Thurs.	Fri.	Sat.	Sun.
MF	SS	AE	SS	MF	SS	AE

Your Custom-Designed Base Period Week

Event/athlete: All athletes.

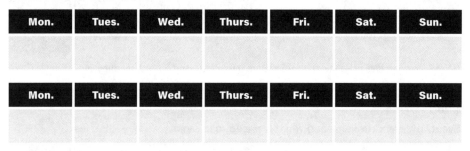

Mon.	Tues.	Wed.	Thurs.	Fri.	Sat.	Sun.

Mon.	Tues.	Wed.	Thurs.	Fri.	Sat.	Sun.

Note: Long-course triathletes, century riders, and ultra-distance riders should lay out a 2-week plan. All other athletes, including recreational and fitness riders, should repeat the standard Base period week.

BUILD

PERIOD LENGTH 8–9 WEEKS

Build Period

Event/athlete: Short-course triathletes, time trialists, recreational and fitness riders.

Mon.	Tues.	Wed.	Thurs.	Fri.	Sat.	Sun.
SS + MF	Recovery	ME (or AnE)	Recovery	ME	Recovery	AE or Event

Note: Recovery rides are done at an easy (zone 1) intensity and for a short duration. In training for very short events lasting less than 1 hour, one of the ME workouts here may be changed to AnE.

Build Period

Event/athlete: Long-course triathletes, century riders, and ultra-distance cyclists.

Mon.	Tues.	Wed.	Thurs.	Fri.	Sat.	Sun.
SS + MF	Recovery	AE	Recovery	ME	Recovery	AE or Event

Note: Recovery rides are done at an easy (zone 1) intensity and for a short duration.

Build Period

Event/athlete: Criteriums and variably paced road races.

Mon.	Tues.	Wed.	Thurs.	Fri.	Sat.	Sun.
SS + MF	Recovery	ME	Recovery	SP + AnE	Recovery	AE or Race

Your Custom-Designed Build Period Week

Mon.	Tues.	Wed.	Thurs.	Fri.	Sat.	Sun.

REST AND RECOVERY

1 WEEK, EVERY 3-4 WEEKS

Rest-and-Recovery Week (in Base and Build Periods)

Event/athlete: All athletes.

Mon.	Tues.	Wed.	Thurs.	Fri.	Sat.	Sun.
MF	Recovery	Recovery	SS	AE	ME (short)	Field Test

Note: These are the same regardless of which of the two periods they are in. They are also quite similar regardless of the rider's purpose or type of event. R&R weeks are not necessary in the Peak and Event periods.

Your Custom-Designed R&R Weeks for the Base and Build Periods

Mon.	Tues.	Wed.	Thurs.	Fri.	Sat.	Sun.

PEAK

PERIOD LENGTH 1–2 WEEKS

Peak Period

Event/athlete: All triathletes and time trialists.

Mon.	Tues.	Wed.	Thurs.	Fri.	Sat.	Sun.
SS + MF	Recovery	AE	ME	Recovery	AE	ME

Note: Recreational and fitness riders who are not doing events do not need to peak and so may omit this period.

Peak Period

Event/athlete: Variably paced events such as road races and criteriums.

Mon.	Tues.	Wed.	Thurs.	Fri.	Sat.	Sun.
SS + MF	Recovery	AE	AnE + ME + SP	Recovery	AE	AnE + MF + SP

Your Custom-Designed Peak Period Week

Mon.	Tues.	Wed.	Thurs.	Fri.	Sat.	Sun.

EVENT

PERIOD LENGTH 1 WEEK

Example of a Training Week for the Event Period

Event/athlete: All triathletes and time trialists.

Mon.	Tues.	Wed.	Thurs.	Fri.	Sat.	Sun.
Recovery	ME (short)	ME (short)	Recovery	ME (very short)	ME (very short)	Event

Note: Recreational and fitness riders not doing an event may omit this period. Workout durations should get shorter during the week, and the number of high-intensity (ME) intervals are also reduced as the week progresses. If the event is on Saturday, move all workouts back one day (for example, Tuesday's workout is done on Monday).

Example of a Training Week for the Event Period

Event/athlete: Variably paced events such as road races and criteriums.

Mon.	Tues.	Wed.	Thurs.	Fri.	Sat.	Sun.
Recovery	AnE + SP (short)	SP (short)	Recovery	AnE (very short)	SP (very short)	Event

Note: If the event is on Saturday, move all workouts back one day (for example, Tuesday's workout is done on Monday).

Your Custom-Designed Event Period Week

Mon.	Tues.	Wed.	Thurs.	Fri.	Sat.	Sun.

Now that you have your weekly plans laid out for the entire season, you have the skeleton of a plan. As you come to each week of the season, all you need to decide is how long the ride will be and how the intensity will be organized. You can get the details for how to organize the session in Chapter 8. As you approach the week on your plan, you'll also want to decide which workouts are best done indoors and which are better suited for an outdoor ride.

With a plan locked in, it's time to get into the details of your week's workouts: how hard (and easy) *you* need to go and for how long, given your current fitness levels and metrics, including heart rate and power.

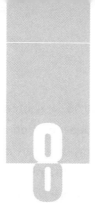

INTENSITY AND
THE INDOOR WORKOUT

As explained in Chapter 6, there are only two components that make up a workout: duration and intensity. It is always these two, whether you are just getting into cycling or have been riding for most of your life. How challenging every workout feels is decided by how long it lasts and how hard the effort is. Duration is the easy part to figure out: You could plan to ride for 1 hour or 90 minutes or some other length of time. You're almost ready to start the ride. But then there is intensity. This is a much trickier decision than choosing duration. This chapter will dig a bit deeper into the intensity of your indoor rides: deciding what the intensity should be for a given workout, reaching the right intensities at the right times, gauging the intensity during the ride, measuring progress using intensity, and optimizing your training time.

SETTING YOUR TRAINING ZONES

Your training zones are the starting place for deciding how hard your ride will be. If you've been with the sport for a few years you know there are several zones, and they were also discussed in Chapter 6. Making this somewhat more complex is that there are two devices you can use to measure intensity on a bike: heart rate monitors and power meters (see Chapter 6 for details). Both have zones unique to them, and both need to be determined. As if that is not enough, there are also many ways to set zones depending on whose training methodology you choose. In this book I'll show you my heart rate zones and Andrew Coggan's power zones. These are two of the most commonly used zone systems, and they match up quite well with the methodology described here. That's not to say you couldn't use someone else's zone system, but it is unlikely to work well with the workouts described in the appendix. Choosing a different zone system means that you would have to modify those workouts, which could be quite a challenge.

HEART RATE ZONES

The starting place for determining your heart rate zones is finding your functional threshold heart rate (FTHR). The test for FTHR is found in the appendix under the "Field Test Main Set" heading. This is a good time to skip ahead to that section and read about the FTHR test. You may even want to do it to determine your threshold (it's a good idea to be rested up for a few days before testing). Remember, your

TABLE 8.1. FTHR Test Results and Training Zones

Heart Rate Zones	Multiply your FTHR of _____ by the percentages below . . .	. . . to determine your personal heart rate zones and record below.
Zone 1	80% and less	
Zone 2	81–89%	
Zone 3	90–93%	
Zone 4	94–99%	
Zone 5a	100–102%	
Zone 5b	103–106%	
Zone 5c	107% and more	

After determining your FTHR with the field test (p. 174), set your heart rate training zones by multiplying your FTHR by the percentage range for each zone, as shown in the middle column. Then record your personal heart rate ranges for each zone in the right-hand column above.

heart rate training zones are specific to the sport you are engaging in. Your running zones, for example, are not applicable to your training in cycling. When you know your FTHR, return to this page and use Table 8.1 to record your zones.

Your heart rate zones are now set. Let's do the same for your power zones.

POWER ZONES

If you have both a heart rate monitor and a power meter, you only need to do the one test you used from the "Field Test Main Set" section of the appendix to establish both your heart rate and power zones. Once you've determined your functional threshold power (FTP), use it to set your power zones by following the guidelines in Table 8.2. This should be done for each power meter you use. For example, if you are riding on a smart trainer, use the power reads from it to determine your FTP. If you then switch back to outdoor riding, you will need to retest your FTP with the power meter that you use on your road bike. Now that you have all of your intensity zones established, let's examine how to use them.

TABLE 8.2. **FTP Test Results and Training Zones**

Power Zones	Multiply your FTP of _____ by the percentages below . . .	. . . to determine your personal power zones and record below.
Zone 1	55% and less	
Zone 2	56–75%	
Zone 3	76–90%	
Zone 4	91–105%	
Zone 5	106–120%	
Zone 6	121–150%	
Zone 7	151% and more	

Determine your power training zones by multiplying your FTP by the percentage range for each zone, as shown below in the middle column (from Allen, Coggan, and McGregor, *Training and Racing with a Power Meter*, 3rd ed.). Then record your personal power zones in the right-hand column above.

SHOULD YOU USE HEART RATE OR POWER ZONES IN WORKOUTS?

As with many questions that have to do with training, the answer starts with "It depends." In this case it depends on what you want to measure when gauging the intensity of your workout: performance or effort. Performance is what you are achieving; effort is how hard you are working. This is an important consideration for understanding what your workouts are all about, so let's dig into it a little deeper.

Remember from earlier that heart rate zones change very little throughout the season even though fitness may change considerably. Rating of perceived exertion (RPE) doesn't change either. An RPE of 7 when you are in poor fitness feels just like an RPE of 7 when you are in great shape. The only thing that changes is how fast you go and how much power you produce at any given heart rate or RPE. As Tour de France winner Greg LeMond once said about becoming more fit, "It doesn't get any easier; you just go faster." That pretty much sums it up.

All of this means that heart rate and RPE are, essentially, measuring the same thing—effort, or how hard you are working. Heart rate is just more precise than the somewhat subjective RPE. Power, in comparison, isn't really measuring effort. Effort doesn't change over time, but performance, measured in power, does change as you become more fit. What power meters tell you is performance, and performance and effort are not the same thing. Here's another way of thinking about this concept: Effort is just another way of saying "input"—what you are experiencing and feeling when you ride a bike. Performance is the "output" you realize as a product of the input. It tells you what you are accomplishing. You may think of this relationship in terms of your car. The tachometer on the car's dashboard tells you how fast the engine is turning—its revolutions per minute. It is not telling you how fast the car is going. The speedometer does that. The tachometer is telling you the engine's effort, or input. The speedometer is telling you performance, or output.

So the answer to the question about which device you should use for a workout—a heart rate monitor or a power meter—is this: If you want to measure effort, use heart rate, and if you want to measure performance, use power.

Most of the workouts you will read about in the appendix are based on power. Here's another way of thinking about this. The lower-intensity workouts intended to boost your aerobic endurance (the AE workouts) are mostly done using heart rate. Recovery rides are also best done using heart rate. Such rides are all about effort. The other workouts, especially the higher-intensity rides, are best done with a power meter.

Since you may not have a power meter (don't forget, there is one on your smart trainer or perhaps your indoor cycle), I also indicate a suggested heart rate for many of the workouts in the appendix. Keep in mind, though, that heart rate monitors are not nearly as effective as power meters for gauging what you are doing in, for example, a high-intensity interval session. And the shorter the high-intensity interval, the less reliable heart rate is. For intervals that are less than about 2 minutes long, assuming you don't have a power meter, you're better off using RPE to gauge intensity (see Figure 6.1) instead of heart rate. Workout RPEs are included in the descriptions in the appendix. Even for longer intervals done above zone 2, you will still have some problems since heart rate rises slowly. This means that for the first couple of minutes, or even longer for the first interval in a set, your heart rate will not be congruent with effort. You therefore have to guess how well you are managing the intensity. Many athletes in this situation pedal very hard to stimulate their heart rates to rise more quickly, and then when it finally reaches the intended level, they reduce the effort. That's actually the opposite of what you should do during a high-intensity interval. It should finish at a higher effort than it started. In fact, doing intervals the other way around leads to the most common problem among racers—poor pacing management. That's one reason why power is the suggested tool for higher-intensity workouts.

INDOOR WORKOUT INTENSITIES

You may recall from Chapter 6 that I suggested having two sets of power zones—one for indoors, and the other for the road. And in the early chapters I described how riding indoors is different from riding outdoors: The movement of the bike is different, and the feel of the "road" is different. All of this adds up to a compromised efficiency that can lead to different power zones. It is important to note that many indoor cycles have flywheels that help to smooth out the ride and simulate the feel of the road more accurately. Most indoor trainers also incorporate a flywheel, with the same anticipated result. Once your zones are set, you are ready to do much the same workouts on your indoor trainer as you would do on the road. It's worth noting here again that you do *not* need two sets of heart rate zones. Heart rate stays the same whether you are indoors or out.

STARTING AND ENDING THE RIDE

Every workout has three parts: the warm-up, the main set, and the cooldown. The main set is the primary purpose of the ride. This could be intervals, a steady ride, hill repeats, skills work, or some combination of these. While the main set is the reason you are doing the ride, preparing for it and returning the body afterward to its normal near-resting state are just as important.

Before getting into the main set, especially if it will be at a high intensity, it's important that you prepare the body for the stress it's about to experience. This preparation is the warm-up.

Sports science research tells us that doing a warm-up, especially before a high-intensity main set, such as intervals or a short race, improves performance. Most of this improvement occurs in the first few minutes of the subsequent high effort. Gradually increasing the warm-up effort without producing fatigue seems to be the best method, according to the studies. The general rule of thumb for warm-up duration is that the shorter the main set intervals are, such as 30-second bursts, the longer the warm-up needs to be. And the opposite is also true: long intervals may be preceded by shorter warm-ups.

The first portion of the warm-up is a very easy, slow turning of the cranks. After a few minutes of getting comfortable on the bike, you can gradually increase the effort to slowly increase your heart rate, breathing, and body temperature. This may be all you need if the ensuing main set is a recovery ride. Warming up before such a ride may only take 5 to 10 minutes.

When warming up before a main set in zone 2 or higher, gradually elevate the heart rate from zone 1 to zone 2 for a couple of minutes. Then return to zone 1 so that you sense a nearly full recovery. After this, do a somewhat harder effort for 2 or 3 minutes. Your heart rate may not respond, but this is normal for early in a workout. Just be sure to briefly achieve an RPE equivalent to what you intend to do in the subsequent main set. This warm-up should only take 10 to 15 minutes and have you ready for the main set to be done at zone 2 or 3.

For an even higher-intensity main set, such as intervals or a race, take a few minutes to raise your RPE briefly to the planned intensity of the main set. If using a power meter, do a few short intensity increases to the goal power for the main set. You may need to do this two or three times with relatively long recoveries between to be ready for the hard main set. Be sure to recover after each hard effort within the warm-up by pedaling slowly. You should feel ready both mentally and physically for the high-intensity main set. The warm-up for a high-intensity main set such as intervals or a race may take 20 minutes, but 30 minutes is not unusual when the main set intensity is quite high.

Properly ending the ride is also important for gradually returning the heart, muscles, breathing mechanisms, and other bodily systems to a low-stress condition. This doesn't need to be highly structured as with the warm-up. It can just be pedaling smoothly and comfortably for several minutes after the main set as the heart rate and breathing return to very low levels.

RECOVERY RIDES

The bulk of all of your rides should be in zone 1. We know what you're thinking: That's too easy; I can go much harder. Although it seems counterintuitive, the research has been telling us since the early 2000s that high levels of fitness are best achieved when around 80 percent of your workouts are done at a very low intensity and at or below the aerobic threshold. The remaining 20 percent of workouts are done above your aerobic threshold, with the largest portion of this at or above the anaerobic or functional threshold. This means that more of your rides should be done in zone 1 than in any other zone. And, of course, your warm-ups and cooldowns should also be largely in zone 1. This heavy emphasis on low intensity with a chunk of the remaining portion done above the functional threshold is known as *polarized training*. The biggest part of your training should be done in zone 1, and heart rate is best for measuring this low intensity. In the appendix, these recovery workouts are found in the "Aerobic Endurance" section.

Not only are recovery rides to be done at a low intensity but they are also best kept to a short duration relative to your other workouts in any given week. Because the purpose is recovery, both intensity and duration should be on the low side.

STEADY RIDES

These are continuous rides done at a relatively constant pace and are very commonly used when trying to improve your aerobic endurance. Steady rides are typically workouts done at about your aerobic threshold in zone 2. Heart rate is the recommended intensity tool for doing these sessions. These steady zone 2 workouts are commonly among the longest rides in a training week since they are quite effective for building aerobic endurance.

Steady rides are also useful for those workouts done in zone 3 in the "Muscular Endurance" section of the appendix. In the early stages of improving your muscular endurance, we recommend relatively long, steady intervals in zone 3, but they are not as long as the zone 2 aerobic threshold workouts. Called "tempo" workouts, these zone 3 intervals are typically around 20 minutes in duration. A power meter is the preferable device for zone 3 rides.

INTERVALS

An interval workout involves dividing the main set into alternating high-intensity and low-intensity segments. While the term "interval" was originally intended to refer to the low-intensity recovery segments between the hard efforts, athletes have come to use the term when referring to the high-intensity portions. It can get a bit confusing. In the appendix we refer to the two portions of the main set as "work intervals" and "recovery intervals" to help clarify.

Such workouts typically are used by athletes when the high-intensity zones are just below the functional threshold (zones 3 and 4) and for those work intervals done above the functional threshold (zones 5, 6, and 7). Power is the preferred intensity-measuring device for these workouts.

It's important to understand that when doing intervals, the recovery portions are just as important as the high-intensity work segments. Sometimes the heart rate will drop to zone 1 during the recovery intervals, although this may not always happen since the recovery intervals are often quite short. The idea here, for most interval workouts, is to achieve only partial recovery before doing the next high-intensity portion. The durations of the recovery intervals are also critical. For example, when doing muscular endurance intervals, the recovery intervals are commonly about one-fourth as long as the work intervals. If you make the recovery intervals longer or you increase their intensity, then the desired workout result may not be realized. For anaerobic endurance interval sessions, the recovery intervals start out early in the season as being equal to the duration of the work intervals—a 1-to-1 ratio. But as the season progresses and anaerobic endurance improves, the recovery intervals gradually are shortened until they are about half the duration of the work intervals—a 2-to-1 ratio. For sprint power workouts, the recovery intervals are always long, usually at least 5 minutes' duration, as it's important to restore the creatine phosphate fuel system that drives such high intensities for very short durations.

The higher the intensity of the main set, the more likely you are to use interval workouts. Interval workouts are therefore found in the "Muscular Endurance," "Anaerobic Endurance," and "Sprint Power" sections of the appendix.

COMBINED-ABILITY WORKOUTS

It's quite common to combine two or more training abilities into a workout's main set. This is common for competitive riders because races often place multiple demands on one's capacity for high-intensity work. A road race or e-race, for example, may involve long climbs done at zone 4 (muscular endurance) followed by attempted breakaways requiring zone 5 (anaerobic endurance) power. Then the finish may involve a very brief, all-out effort (sprint power). During the Build period of the season, such workouts may well be a necessity for race preparation. For the fitness rider, the combined-ability workout provides an opportunity for training variety in addition to stronger riding when encountering different situations when on the road, such as headwinds and tailwinds, climbing and descending, catching up to a group, or just alternating hard and easy rides for the fun of it.

MEASURING PROGRESS WITH INTENSITY

How do you know if you are becoming more fit? The most common indication is how you feel during long or high-intensity rides. But that's quite subjective and may vary from day to day based on your fatigue level, sleep status, mental stress, or any number of other lifestyle variables. A more objective way of determining changes in fitness uses the workout data from your heart rate monitor and power meter. The other intensity metric examined in this chapter is RPE. But, of course, it can't help you determine whether you are becoming more fit or not since it also is subjective. Heart rate and power are the only objective intensity metrics available to you. And they are giving you such feedback with every ride. The "tachometer" and "speedometer" are always telling you how you are feeling and how you are performing. For measuring how you are progressing as a rider, we need to look at both heart rate and power.

EFFICIENCY FACTOR

In any aspect of life, such as managing a business, driving your car, or riding a bike, whenever you can identify both input and output, you can then know something called *efficiency*. Similar to economy, efficiency is the cost of production or accomplishment—how much input is needed to produce a given output. The mathematical formula for efficiency is output divided by input. If we apply this formula to training on a bicycle, we get power divided by heart rate. This number tells you how efficient you are when riding a bike. In the language of endurance sports, efficiency is "aerobic fitness." In other words, the more power (output) you can produce at a given heart rate (input), the greater your aerobic fitness. Note that this is not *anaerobic* fitness because the formula doesn't work as precisely when you are riding above your functional threshold.

What we are therefore looking to see happen as your aerobic fitness increases is that you produce more power at any given heart rate. Simple enough. Over time this number, called the *efficiency factor* (EF), should rise when comparing similar types of workouts. So, how do you know your fitness is improving? If the EF number is generally rising over several weeks, you are becoming more efficient, meaning more aerobically fit. Having both a heart rate monitor and power meter allows you to precisely measure how your aerobic fitness is progressing. How cool is that?

FUNCTIONAL THRESHOLD POWER

Another great indicator of fitness is your functional threshold power (FTP). If it is rising, you are becoming more fit—and more powerful. You'll know if this is happening if you test your FTP every 4 to 6 weeks throughout the season following the test guidelines described in appendix. A rising FTP is a sure sign of greater fitness. But, even if your FTP is not increasing, you could still be improving your fitness because heart rate may be lower at sub-FTP intensities.

There are other ways of measuring fitness progression using a power meter, such as "time to exhaustion" and "stamina." But these are rather complex metrics requiring power-analysis software for your computer called WKO (available at trainingpeaks.com) and are beyond the scope of this book.

OPTIMIZING YOUR TRAINING TIME

Whether you are a recreational, fitness, or performance rider, the biggest challenge to becoming more fit is time. If you only had a couple more hours per week to ride, you could definitely improve your fitness. But you've got a lot going on in your life besides riding a bike. There's your family, which comes first; your career, which is also highly important; and a multitude of other demands on your time.

You squeeze bike workouts in whenever you can, but it isn't always easy. The more stuff you have in your life, the harder it becomes to become as fit as you'd like. What can be done about that? How can you make the best use of the limited time you have available in order to achieve your fitness goal?

POLARIZATION

I've already mentioned this once in this chapter, but it bears repeating here. The key to increasing your fitness is to divide the intensity of your workouts into three categories: below the aerobic threshold, above the anaerobic threshold, and between the two thresholds (see Figure 6.2). By far most training should be in zone 1. That's in the neighborhood of 70 to 80 percent of your workouts. Perhaps the biggest mistake eager riders make is doing too much at moderate to high intensities. To get the most benefit from these hard workouts, you need to come into them physically and mentally fresh. If you try to do this several times each week, the quality—and fitness benefits—of these hard workouts will be compromised. Performing the hard workouts only 2 or, at most, 3 times in a week, with the others being recovery rides or days off, means you'll be ready and eager when it's time to go hard again.

DOSE

If you take my advice of doing only two or three high-intensity workouts in a week, there are still a couple considerations to make the most of those rides.

The first concern is the "dose" of the hard workouts. This simply means how hard you make it. The human body, yours included, is not a machine that can operate at a high level of work without breaking down. We all have limits, and it's best to exceed those limits by only small amounts. If you did three very hard intervals last week and you felt empowered but somewhat tired afterward, do not do six of the same intervals this week. That's going to be too much. The dose is too great. You'd be taking a big risk that could cause your knee to become inflamed, or you'd be too tired to even do a recovery ride the next day, or you may find it hard to sleep the night after that ride.

Your body has limits, but it also has a remarkable capacity to grow stronger and more fit when the doses increase only slightly over time. Making a big jump in the intensity of your workout may seem like the thing to do in the moment, especially if your friend is doing it. But it's seldom the right thing to do. If the dose is too great and the body becomes overly fatigued, you are unlikely to reap the full benefits of the workout. It's not just that that single workout is wasted; it also drags down the quality or quantity of subsequent rides. You may actually lose fitness by making one workout too hard.

DENSITY

Similar to dose is density. This has to do with how closely spaced your hard workouts are. Get them too close together, and you're likely to shortchange the benefits because the body simply doesn't have enough time to adapt, which I'll get back to shortly. How should they be spaced? Let's take a look at a couple of examples.

Imagine you are planning to do two high-intensity workouts in a week. One of them is muscular endurance intervals and the other is anaerobic endurance intervals. These are both very hard workouts. And they require a good deal of recovery time afterward. The worst thing you could do is schedule these two rides on subsequent days, such as on Tuesday and Wednesday. The second ride is sure to be a downer. You won't get much from it because of fatigue. Furthermore, you also now have six days until the next hard workout on the following Tuesday. That means you are highly likely to lose any fitness gains you may have achieved with the back-to-back workouts. Remember the principle in sports science called "reversibility," which was described in Chapter 7. It means that if the wait between workouts is too long, fitness is lost. How long should the break between hard workouts be to avoid reversibility? It should probably be no more than 72 to 96 hours. That's three or four days. An occasional five-day break may be OK. But a regular diet of five-day breaks between hard rides is sure to prove counterproductive.

What would be a good way to space two hard workouts? If they were done on Wednesday and Saturday, there would be a three-day and a four-day interruption in intense training, making for an optimal routine and a near-perfect density when only doing two high-intensity workouts in a week. The other three to five days that you may train would then involve recovery rides, which, in all, would make for a nearly perfect polarized week.

Three days of hard training in a week—for example, on Tuesdays, Thursdays, and Saturdays—would also make for a well-balanced training week. But you'd have to decide if the dose is too great with this pattern.

ADAPTATION

How does fitness come about? Most riders think it is the direct result of hard workouts. That's only right to a certain extent. Hard workouts only create the *potential* for greater fitness. You don't become stronger on a bike by just doing hard rides. It takes more than that. The other slice of the fitness pie is sleep because this is actually when fitness gains occur. When you're asleep, especially in deep sleep, your body releases hormones that cause the tissues in your body— muscles, bones, nerves, and more—to grow stronger. The body adapts and grows more fit during sleep.

So, what happens if you do a hard workout one day and then shorten your sleep cycle that night in order to fit more into your life? You don't fully reap the benefits of the hard workout. You simply wasted a sizeable chunk of the day's ride.

How do you determine how much sleep you should get? You need to attain deep sleep a few times each night in order to adapt to the stress of a hard workout. This usually means that a rider needs between 7 and 9 hours of sleep each night to get the most from their training time. Are you regularly getting that much sleep? If not, something needs to give. Your life is too busy, or you're not prioritizing sleep. If your goal is to become more fit, remember that doing hard workouts is not enough. Sleep will help you become more fit and will also improve almost every other important aspect of your life, from health to body weight, mental concentration, and so much more.

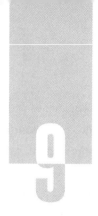

PUTTING IT ALL TOGETHER

The best thing about being fit is using that hard-earned fitness. This book is focused on riding inside, but on a grander scale, fitness opens up a world of opportunities. You are not a laboratory rat, and training is not a science experiment. You're an athlete, and while we can use sports science and power data to guide the progression of training and increase the precision of performance analysis, you are not training for the sake of improving numbers on piece of paper. You're training to become more capable, to increase your capacity for work so you can go farther, faster, and longer than you could before.

Sometimes your work is aimed at optimizing performance for a specific competition, but in the grand scheme of things, being a lifelong athlete means maintaining a broad enough base of fitness that you can say yes to jumping into any activity that sounds fun or has to be done. You may be a competitive cyclist or triathlete, but you should be able to play a pickup game of basketball or baseball without being sore for a week. You should be able to move furniture or do yardwork without injuring yourself. And you should be able to jump on your bike and take on challenges outside the narrow scope of your competitive goals. Instead of limiting yourself to being a bike racer or triathlete, broaden your perspective and aim to be an athlete who happens to race a bike or compete in triathlons.

Now that you have gained all this fitness and power riding inside, it's time to put it to good use. You can jump into e-races and test yourself against riders from around the globe without leaving home. You can take your riding outside and go to the local group ride or register for all manner of cycling or triathlon events. And it is also important to realize that it's not a binary choice; integrating indoor and outdoor cycling—along with other activities—is perhaps the most effective way to create a winning training plan. So, now that you have built up your fitness by riding inside, let's see how to make the most of it.

INTEGRATING INDOOR AND OUTDOOR TRAINING FOR BEST RESULTS

Cyclists and triathletes have always struggled to find time to ride because of the logistical hurdles of aligning the available time with daylight hours, a place to ride, and the equipment necessary. Expanding the ways we can ride inside opens up available training time many athletes thought they'd never see again. The key is combining indoor and outdoor riding, as well as combining different types of indoor cycling, into a cohesive plan.

FREQUENCY

The most common question about structuring training across the various types of indoor cycling is how frequently an athlete should do structured workouts versus free rides/group rides or e-races and unstructured sufferfests. First, go back and review the material in Chapter 8 on dose and density of training. How you structure the doses of training and the amount of time between them will depend on your current fitness, your training and competition goals, and the amount of stress in your daily life. A good starting point is to make time for two (maybe three) structured workout sessions per week, at least one of which should be focused on muscular endurance.

For athletes who are training to peak for a specific event or short time period within a season, I recommend limiting e-races and unstructured hard rides to once per week. The intensity of these sessions can be very high, which is great for accumulating time at very high power outputs and for learning how to handle repeated efforts at unpredictable times. They also necessitate a substantial amount of recovery before you can execute another high-quality structured workout. Goal-oriented athletes make the most progress through structured interval training, so when balancing out your schedule for the week it is wise to prioritize purposeful workouts over sessions that are hard for the sake of being hard. If you are training for anything other than time trials or triathlons, incorporate more e-races and hard, unpredictable virtual group rides as your event nears in order to make your training more specific to the variable demands of racing.

So, if there are one or two structured workouts and one e-race/sufferfest, that leaves potentially four to five additional days in the week. Two or three of them should be rest days or easy recovery rides, and the others should be zone 2 aerobic endurance rides, which can be solo rides inside or out, or group rides outdoors or via interactive apps.

THE BEST INDOOR OPTIONS FOR SPECIFIC WORKOUTS

As you'll recall from Chapter 7, workouts are designed to target either basic or advanced abilities—or a combination of both. To review, the six abilities are:

Aerobic endurance (AE)
Speed skills (SS)
Muscular force (MF)
Muscular endurance (ME)
Anaerobic endurance (AnE)
Sprint power (SP)

You can train all six abilities while riding inside, and to make the most of your training, you can align the ability you're training with the type of indoor cycling that is best suited for it.

Aerobic Endurance (AE)

Recovery rides and aerobic threshold rides can certainly be done alone, but having virtual company through an interactive app can be helpful. A lot of riders skip recovery rides indoors because it seems like a waste of time to get on an indoor trainer just to go easy. But indoors or outdoors, recovery rides serve an important purpose and, for the highly experienced rider, are better for your training progression than not riding at all. Getting together with a club or a friend through an interactive indoor cycling app can provide the incentive necessary to get on the bike. Having company can also help keep your easy ride easy. Riding too hard during a recovery ride is a mistake coaches see all the time, and peer pressure from a group is a good way to enforce the "go easy" mantra.

Aerobic threshold rides tend to be your long rides of the week. These are zone 2 rides at a conversational pace or the zone 2 portion of a combined ride where you might spend an hour at aerobic threshold and include a speed skills or muscular force set in the middle. Long zone 2 rides outdoors are great to do solo and can certainly be done solo indoors, but many riders find them more enjoyable when connected to apps that feature video and virtual courses, or with groups through interactive apps. It may be difficult to find long aerobic threshold rides at indoor cycling studios, however, because "moderate and steady" isn't very marketable.

Speed Skills (SS)

You can sneak these cadence and pedal-stroke drills into interactive virtual group rides or even during live indoor cycling classes. It's just a matter of changing your focus and perhaps your gearing or resistance. Whether you're riding inside alone or with a group, you have to reduce the resistance on the trainer to accomplish these drills, particularly spin-ups and 9-to-3 drills. Riding in erg mode on a virtual course makes this difficult because the trainer is setting the resistance based on your weight and the grade of the virtual course. You can either do them on a virtual descent when the resistance lightens up or switch your smart trainer to level mode and reduce the resistance manually. With old-school trainers, shifting into a light gear will do the trick because even with a high cadence, you'll be at the low end of the trainer's power curve. A more advanced version of spin-ups and 9-to-3s is to ride with a high cadence at zone 4 because the end goal of working on your pedal stroke is being able to pedal quickly at high power outputs.

The isolated-leg drills are often executed better indoors than outdoors. If you are using your bike on a stationary trainer, you can either unclip and rest your foot on a stool or stable part of the trainer or stay clipped in and just let the "resting" leg go around. The point of the isolated drill is to feel and minimize the "dead spots" at the top and bottom of the pedal stroke. Without the power of the opposing leg, you'll notice how little force you exert from about 11 o'clock to 1 o'clock and after the 5 o'clock position. As with the 9-to-3 drill with both feet, aim to kick your foot across the top of the stroke and pull through the bottom of the stroke when pedaling with one foot.

Muscular Force (MF)

Flat force and hill force intervals are short efforts (6–8 pedal strokes for each leg) that require high torque to accelerate against heavy resistance. For indoor training, these are best done alone or in a specific group workout where everyone performs the same workout. They are harder to do during an interactive group ride. If you have a smart trainer with a "level" setting, increase the level so the power curve starts out high. Otherwise, you are more likely to spin up too quickly before encountering sufficiently heavy resistance. Riders with rear-wheel or direct-drive trainers with fluid or wind resistance will need to start in a large gear. If you have a magnetic resistance unit on a specialized indoor cycle, like a Peloton, you'll have to increase the resistance significantly so you have substantial resistance to getting the freewheel moving. You don't have to start from an absolute standing start, but you want the cranks to be moving very slowly to start the intervals.

Muscular Endurance (ME)

Tempo, cruise, and sweet spot intervals are among the most common intensities you'll see in preplanned structured workouts in indoor cycling apps. These intensities can also be pretty easily incorporated into virtual group rides on interactive apps even if it's a free ride rather than a structured workout. Because the interval durations for muscular endurance ability workouts range from 6 to 20 minutes at specific power outputs (see Chapter 7), they are well suited for erg mode or a manual resistance setting at a target power output. If you are just looking to accumulate time at intensity, erg mode works great for these efforts. When you are looking to transition your riding to outdoor training and events, it is important to spend some time doing these intervals on level mode or on a virtual course so you can learn the pacing and motivation necessary to reach and hold the appropriate effort.

Anaerobic Endurance (AnE)

VO_2max intervals, pyramid intervals, and group ride work is what indoor cycling setups do best. The VO_2max intervals and pyramid intervals feature short efforts of 30 seconds to 3 minutes and a total work time of 3 to 15 minutes. The intensity of the efforts is power zone 5 or an RPE of 9 out of 10. Erg mode on a smart trainer is not the best way to execute these intervals because the point is for you to reach and maintain the highest power output you can sustain for the duration of each interval. It is better to use the level mode on a smart trainer for these or rely on the power curve of a fluid or wind resistance unit.

With magnetic resistance units on dedicated indoor cycles, the only complication is that you need to manually increase the resistance level to start the interval and then manually reduce the resistance for recovery periods. When the intervals and recovery periods are extremely short (30-second efforts with 30-second recoveries, for instance), that can get difficult to keep up with—especially as you fatigue from the efforts.

When I want an athlete to truly give everything they have during VO_2max intervals or pyramid intervals, I make them execute the workout indoors for their own safety. If you really go all-out for five 3-minute VO_2max intervals, you will be gasping for breath and have nothing left at the end. I'd rather a cyclist or triathlete close their eyes, drop their head, and hunch over the handlebars on an indoor trainer than have them do that on a road or trail. To compete outdoors, you will need to be able to control the bike while exerting that much effort, but during the process of training, indoors is the safest place for max effort intervals.

Virtual group rides, e-races, and in-person live cycling classes are other logical places for anaerobic endurance work. Depending on the app settings, one of the benefits of virtual group rides and in-person classes is that you can't get dropped, so you don't have to hold anything back. In the real world, athletes almost always hold a little bit of power in reserve so they have something left in the tank to avoid getting left behind after their city limit sprint or hard pull on the front of the group. Many cyclists who compete in e-races note they are often more difficult than any real-world race they competed in, and the lack of risk—either from crashing or being physically left behind—may play a role in allowing riders to reach higher power outputs and sustain them longer.

Sprint Power (SP)

Sprint power main sets—form sprints, jumps, and group sprints—can be tricky on rear-wheel and direct-drive trainers because of cyclists' tendencies to swing the bike side-to-side while driving downward with each pedal stroke. When the bike has a stable and immovable base, your movement on top of the bike won't be as effective and can be counterproductive. However, there are benefits to sprinting indoors. Just like riding an indoor trainer can help you correct a choppy pedal stroke, sprinting on an indoor trainer can help you deliver power to the pedals with less side-to-side movement.

Group sprint workouts can be accomplished with a structured workout in an interactive app, more informally during a group ride or e-race, and as part of in-person live cycling classes. When it comes to real-world racing it is important, however, to spend time practicing sprints with other riders close by. Not only do you need real-world sprint practice to learn how to gauge the timing and intensity of your efforts, but you also need to be comfortable in the close quarters of a group ride or racing situation. At the end of an outdoor race, you have to pick your line, maneuver with the riders around you, and keep yourself and everyone else safe.

Particularly as athletes get older, training should shift to increase emphasis on generalized strength and cardiovascular fitness and decrease emphasis on sport-specific performance. It's not that competitive goals are less valuable to aging athletes or that specificity is less effective. It's that generalized conditioning is necessary to maintain the strength, mobility, and balance to prevent injuries that would otherwise take you off the field of play.

Who is an "aging athlete?" For simplicity's sake let's assume that's anyone over the age of 50. While I've known many half-century athletes who are still successfully competing with 30-somethings, by this stage of life most of us start to see things change a bit. The most obvious is the need for more recovery time following hard workouts and races. Athletes in their 20s can manage several hard days in a row and still perform at a high level each time. Aging athletes need more rest-and-recovery time now than we did a few years ago. As the years pile up, we notice other changes. Here are three that I've found have a lot to do with maintaining performance as we move beyond 50.

Other than recovery, the most obvious change is that aerobic capacity (VO_2max) begins to noticeably decline. You breathe just as hard on long hard efforts as you have always done, but you aren't going as fast or the power isn't as great. This happens gradually. It more than likely started in your mid-30s and continued into your 40s, but perhaps wasn't really noticeable then because you had become a smarter racer and knew how to take advantage of your other strengths. But usually by your 50th birthday, you're aware of it. This is normal. It happens to all of us. And short of a magic wand, I don't know of any way to completely reverse the trend. But you can temporarily reverse it—perhaps. To do this, you slow the decline of your VO_2max. By this point in life, most of us start gravitating toward long, slow distance. Other than an occasional all-out effort, usually in a race or hard group ride, we find it somewhat more comfortable to focus on duration at the expense of intensity (although workout duration has been shown to decrease with aging also). We become focused on how many miles or hours we're doing rather than how hard the rides are. To boost your VO_2max you need to reverse that trend. To do that I suggest including two types of workouts in your weekly training. Both should be high-intensity intervals done at near or above your anaerobic threshold. In the appendix you'll find guidelines in two categories that will fit the bill—muscular endurance and anaerobic endurance workouts.

The second change that begins to appear after 50 is a loss of muscle mass. Again, this doesn't happen suddenly but also helps explain, in part, the decline in VO_2max because the more sport-specific muscle you have, the more oxygen you can process. Unfortunately, this slide happens because we get lazy. We hire someone to cut the grass or clean the house. We're less inclined to ride hilly courses or push to our limits. Or we stop going to the gym . . . The bottom line is that if you don't stress your muscles, they are lost. Use it or lose it. The fix? Make it a point to stress the muscles at least twice each week—every week. Perhaps the best way to do that is by getting back to the gym. As a cyclist, the muscles you are most concerned about are the ones in your legs that drive the ankles, knees, and hips when pedaling. You already know the best exercises: squats, leg press, lunges, or any weight-loaded exercise that causes you to extend the ankles, knees, and hips at the same time. Don't like going to the gym? I understand. So go to the muscular force section of the appendix to find on-the-bike alternatives. Then do them regularly.

The third change is one we're all too familiar with—an increase in body fat. Part of the reason we gain fat with aging is that our anabolic hormones, such as testosterone, estrogen, human growth hormone, insulin-like growth factor, and many, many more are in serious decline by age 50. And what stimulates the production of these tissue-building hormones? High-intensity exercise, such as intervals and weight lifting. But hormone production doesn't happen during the hard ride or gym session. Those only create the potential for the hormones to do their thing. The actual changes that take place in the body mostly happen while sleeping. That's something most of us don't get enough of. We try to wedge too many things into our days. Where do we nearly always find that "extra" time to do more stuff? By reducing bed time. Because of this, I tell athletes with the most ambitious goals in sport that they can only have three things in their lives—family, career, and training. All of the other stuff must go. I know those other things are important to you. But there's only one you. It really just comes down to how badly you want to achieve your athletic goal. Your call.

You have choices to make every day. I've suggested a few of them here that have the potential to improve your cycling performance despite aging. It's up to you to decide which, if any, you will do.

TAKING INDOOR FITNESS OUTDOORS

Riding inside can build all the fitness you need to perform at your best in outdoor events. There's no doubt cyclists or triathletes can accomplish all of the high-intensity interval work their outdoor-only counterparts would normally do throughout the year. But particularly with the current focus on polarized training and reverse periodization, high-intensity interval work is typically only 10–20 percent of an athlete's total annual workload. The other 80+ percent is low- to moderate-intensity endurance riding, and that's the harder part to replicate entirely indoors. With the emergence of Zwift and other interactive apps, "free riding" at an endurance pace is more appealing than it used to be, and the rise of e-racing is making it possible to feed your competitive drive without riding outside.

Most cyclists and triathletes, however, are training indoors with the intent to participate or compete in events outdoors. The most common scenario is using a mixture of indoor and outdoor training sessions to maximize your available training time. More and more, the percentage of overall training being completed indoors is growing, and training primarily indoors can have both positive and negative impacts on outdoor performance.

The advantage of indoor fitness is the level of control we have over the amount and distribution of intensity. If you want precision in training, you can't beat riding structured workouts indoors on a smart trainer in erg mode. At the end of a week or a month of training, your power files and training data will be close to perfect because your motivation and willpower played no part in determining your performance. As I have mentioned before, this is also a significant disadvantage to training indoors with erg mode, because you risk losing or not developing the internal drive and expertise for self-pacing.

ON-THE-ROAD EXPERIENCE

Perfect training files don't necessarily equate to optimal preparation for real-world cycling performances. In the Dark Ages, when cyclists and triathletes only rode indoors when they absolutely needed to, the transition back to outdoor group rides and races was pretty seamless. The outdoor skills might have gotten a bit rusty but came back quickly. Now that athletes are spending more and more time riding inside (and building tremendous fitness indoors), there has been a significant dissociation between fitness and skill.

If you have spent hours and hours on a smart trainer or plugged in to Zwift, The Sufferfest, TrainerRoad, Rouvy, FulGaz, or any of the other indoor cycling apps, you may very well have the fitness and power to ride in an outdoor peloton at 30 mph. To be successful and safe in that environment, however, you need the handling skills to ride shoulder to shoulder at that speed, to brake appropriately before corners, and to take good lines through turns. Without those skills, it's like putting a bunch of brand-new drivers into Ferraris and having them go out on the track with people who have been driving Ferraris for 10 years. Everyone on the track has similar horsepower, but only some know how to drive the car.

For decades, cycling skill and speed developed side by side (for the most part) because beginners didn't have the power to keep up with experienced riders who had gradually learned how to go fast over the same timeframe they gained fitness. Riders learned the skills necessary to handle higher speeds as they gained the power required to achieve those speeds. For some athletes who primarily ride inside, that process has been upended and is causing some unintended—and dangerous—consequences.

Preparation for Time Trialing and Triathlons

Aerodynamics is one of the most important aspects of racing for triathletes and time trialers. On an indoor trainer you can sit upright to increase power. But in triathlon and time trialing outside, you know that is a grave mistake. Any gains made from a more powerful upright position on the bike will cost much more energy than being fully aero. When training inside for such events, it's critical that you ride a bike that is intended for your type of event and that you assume a fully aerodynamic position when doing high-intensity, race-like workouts. Your power numbers may be somewhat less impressive, but you'll be better prepared when it's race day. For easy, aerobic rides, any bike will do.

It's also important for competitive triathletes to train in a way that is similar to what they will experience in a race. While it may be fun to do an e-race, that's really not what triathlon is about. Triathlon is a relatively steady intensity from beginning to end with climbing and descending hills as the only time power significantly increases and decreases. That's exactly the opposite from what you would experience in an e-race. While it may be fun to occasionally do an e-race, a steady diet of these will be counterproductive to your triathlon race goals. While this may seem counterintuitive, the physiological gains made from doing highly variably paced road races does not cross over to better steady-intensity racing.

Learn and Practice in Group Rides

Teaching handling skills is beyond the scope of this book, but if you are relatively new to outdoor road racing, it is important to spend time learning how to draft, ride in close quarters comfortably, hold a straight line while looking back or taking a drink, and line up for a corner and adjust your speed. Easy-paced and endurance-focused group rides are great for working on the basics because the speeds are lower, there is less competitiveness between riders for position in the pack, and you will have enough power that you don't need to worry about losing contact with the group if you let a gap open up temporarily.

Strong novices often rely too heavily on power to avoid uncomfortable situations. When you are going to a group ride or training race with the intention of improving your skills and confidence, you have to resist the temptation to just use your power output to throttle your way out of trouble. You may have the power to ride to the side of the group and keep up without drafting, but what you need are the skills to read the wind direction, find the best drafting position, and ride within inches of the wheel ahead of you. Similarly, you might be strong enough to close big gaps, but you need the skills to prevent those gaps from opening in the first place.

Learn to Win Before Upgrading

In addition to handling skills, it is crucial for competitive road racers to learn *how to race* and how to win in the novice categories before upgrading to the more advanced categories. Moving up into more competitive fields too quickly is one of the biggest mistakes cyclists make. The tactical lessons about how to stay in a good position within the peloton, how to form a breakaway, where to attack the group, how to follow the right wheels, and how to launch a winning sprint are learned through repetition.

When the speed and intensity of the race are well within your capabilities, you can focus on tactics and decision-making. In the course of a one-hour race, you could try forming a breakaway five times, sprint for three primes and the finale, and go from riding at the front to bringing up the rear and everywhere in between. When athletes move up too quickly, they have fewer opportunities to learn because they have to spend more mental and physical energy to just keep up. Develop winning skills first, and then you'll be able to execute them in the final lap of an elite criterium.

Beat Them at Their Own Game

Horsepower and the ability to sustain an unrelenting pace are the primary advantages inside riders have when they take their fitness outdoors. Your potential weaknesses, however, are equally well-known to the riders you are up against. If power data were the only determinant for winning races, we could just compare power profiles and hand out checks. In reality, underpowered riders can and often do win races by making objectively stronger cyclists waste energy. If you are primarily an inside rider, watch out for the following tactics competitors will try using against you:

- **Surges.** Many inside riders are great at maintaining a fast and steady pace, like a locomotive. You're accustomed to tapping out a consistent rhythm, knowing exactly how long efforts will be and when it's time to increase or decrease power output. To beat you, competitors will try to disrupt your rhythm and make you respond to repeated surges. Each time you accelerate to go after them, you're burning another match or firing another bullet, and their goal is to leave you empty-handed before the finale.

Solution: *In training be sure to incorporate indoor and outdoor workouts that feature rapid and frequent changes in intensity. Participate in e-races, group rides, and training races so you learn to initiate and respond to repeated hard efforts at random intervals and separated by variable periods of recovery. In competition, be patient and discerning about the accelerations you follow. Your strength is the ability to sustain a high pace, so use that to reel in attackers rather than always bolting after them.*

- **Letting you do the work.** When you spend most of your time riding indoors on your own—even if you are technically riding with a group via an interactive app—you are used to doing all the work yourself. Even with drafting in Zwift, there is no change in the resistance you feel through your smart trainer; the effect only changes the behavior of your avatar. Outdoors, experienced riders take advantage of inexperienced athletes' desires to prove themselves by leaving you on the front of the group or paceline as long as you're willing to stay there. Pulling on the front is also the least complicated thing to do, so strong riders with less experience often feel more comfortable and confident just staying there. For the group, it's a great way to save energy and wear you down, so when the time comes, they can leave you behind with a few strong accelerations.

Solution: *Do your share of the pace making or chasing and then pull off to the side and drift back to get into the draft. If you are in a paceline, be sure you save a little something so you can get on the wheel at the back of the line. There is no award for the rider who does the most work and then gets dropped.*

- **Hanging you out in the wind.** Savvy outdoor riders will try to take advantage of the wind and maneuver you into positions where they are in the draft and you are not. If you are less comfortable in a pack, it is likely you will ride close to the sides of the field rather than right in the heart of it. When you're riding out on the edge of the group, it is relatively easy for someone next to you to pressure you off the wheel and out into the wind. If you are not good at reading the wind direction, you may also find yourself on the wrong side when the group turns into a crosswind.

  Solution: *Work on getting comfortable moving around in the field. The peloton is a dynamic environment, and you have to be able to move side to side and back to front within it. There is no perfect place to be because the perfect place is always changing. If you get bumped out into the wind or misread the wind direction, the best thing to do is recognize it quickly and find a way to get back into the draft right away.*

- **Pressuring you through technical features.** This tactic is most clearly visible on climbs and technical descents. Riding inside and participating in e-races gives riders the power to climb like a rocket, but outdoors getting to the summit with the lead group is only half the battle. If you can't ride down the mountain confidently and safely, you will be minutes behind by the time you get to the bottom. Even worse, you'll be caught by riders who were several minutes slower than you on the climb, and they may not have the power to help you get back to the lead group. Once competitors know they can leave you behind—or catch you—when the road or trail gets technical, they know how to beat you. And they don't have to drop you all at once. If you have to accelerate harder out of every corner because you're taking slower lines or hitting the brakes more, they'll keep up that pressure to wear you down faster.

Solution: *Practice handling skills. People take ski lessons to get better at skiing and golf lessons to improve their swing, but endurance athletes tend to rely on experience and observation to pick up skills rather than actual lessons. Work with a skills coach who has domain expertise in the cycling discipline you're trying to master. A weekend skills camp can save you years of trial and error, start you out with solid fundamentals you can build on, and give you tools to take your skills and confidence to the next level. If you had skills when you were younger and you're returning to the peloton with a more mature perspective on risk, a refresher course is a great way to rediscover confidence in your handling skills.*

RACING INSIDE: A GUIDE TO E-RACING

Whoever invented the wheel probably used it to have a race against the second person who made one. Humans thrive on competition, so it should be no surprise that riders using interactive indoor cycling apps quickly found ways to create e-races. With the ever-increasing challenges and costs of putting on real-world races, e-racing offers a cost-effective way to bring together cyclists from all over the world for competitions. When the 2020 cycling season was put on hold due to the COVID-19 pandemic, e-racing surged in popularity. Professional cycling teams that needed a way to connect with fans and meet sponsor obligations started online group rides and banded together with other teams to create virtual races. The egalitarian nature of e-racing allows amateurs to enter races with the pros, race at almost any time of day or night, and race against riders from all over the world.

As of spring 2020, Zwift is the primary e-racing app for cyclists. While there are a few other apps that can accommodate e-racing, Zwift's membership numbers and the numbers of riders and teams racing on Zwift dwarf the other alternatives. As a result, the specifics and tactics discussed below are based on the experience of Zwift e-races, although many of the concepts will apply equally well for e-races on other platforms.

E-races work a lot like any other race in the real world. Once you select a race, based on the course and your category (more on that in a bit), you are put in a virtual start corral. When the race begins, your position in the peloton is tracked in real time as your avatar moves through the field. By using your power wisely, you can stay near the front of the pack, sit in and draft, attack off the front, form breakaways, and split the field, and you can sprint for the win. You can also get dropped, be caught behind a split, or drift too far back in the pack and take yourself out of contention.

There are also some unique aspects of e-racing that will be new to anyone with an outdoor racing background. In Zwift races, riders are randomly awarded "PowerUps," which among other things can provide an extra aero advantage or reduce your weight for short periods of time. Racers also have to learn new methods for reading a race. In real-world racing, you can see when riders are at their limits by reading their body language and facial expressions, observing how they are pedaling or moving on the bike, and listening to changes in their breathing. With the rare exception of e-races contested in a live environment or with video conferencing, you can't see the riders you're up against in an e-race. You'll be able to see their current watts per kilogram (W/kg), but not their height, weight, or actual watts per kilogram at FTP. And without context it is hard to know whether they can sustain a particular effort or are about to crack.

Though e-racing is relatively new, there are some fundamental tactics and strategies you can use to improve your performance.

CHOOSE THE RIGHT RACE FOR YOU

If you are riding a smart trainer, the resistance you feel is set according to your height (taller riders have more aerodynamic drag), weight, and the grade of the course. This means that lightweight riders still have a power-to-weight advantage over heavy riders when going uphill, and that heavier riders still have an advantage going downhill and on the flats where they produce greater absolute power. E-races are held on a variety of courses, from flat routes to punchy climbs to mountain passes. Some courses consist of many laps on a short course,

Back in Chapter 3 we discussed the various types of indoor cycling equipment and technologies and how they work together. To get to the start line for an e-race, here are the tools you need and steps to take.

1. **Interactive app and account.** Whether you are using Zwift, Rouvy, RGT Cycling, or another app, you'll need an account and have the app downloaded to a phone, tablet, laptop, or Apple TV, depending on the platforms available. And here's a tip: Use a big screen. Workouts and free rides are workable with a small phone screen or a laptop a few feet away, but e-racing works better with a bigger screen because you have to be able to see the data and observe other avatars quickly while you are going hard. If you need to use the app on a smaller device, stream the content from your device to a larger screen.

2. **Power measurement.** To compete in an e-race, you need a way to transmit your power output into the app. A smart trainer is the most straightforward way to do it. Open the app, turn on the trainer, and pair the two. If you are using a classic trainer or rollers, you will need a bicycle-mounted power meter that directly measures power (as opposed to calculating power from wind and accelerometers). Pair the power meter to the app via Bluetooth. If you have an older power meter that only transmits ANT+, you will need a special dongle or a converter. Many apps have a virtual power feature that uses a speed sensor and a classic trainer's known power curve to calculate your power. But because it is not a direct measure of power, many e-races won't accept virtual power.

3. **Heart rate monitor.** Many e-races require the use of a heart rate monitor to provide context for your power output and discover riders who are either deliberately cheating or using poorly calibrated power meters or trainers.

4. **Get registered.** Entering an e-race is easy. There's no packet pickup, no race numbers to pin, and no per-race entry fee (the entry fee is your subscription to the app). For e-racing on Zwift, there are two additional one-time steps. Connect your Zwift account to Zwiftpower.com and a Strava account and

agree to share data with both. Zwiftpower.com is a community-driven site that generates race results, and some e-race organizers use Strava data to flag riders or catch cheaters. If your Strava data says you've never sustained more than 3 watts/kg on a climb and you're pumping out 5 watts/kg on Zwift, something's not right.

5. **Get connected and ready.** Get on the bike and start spinning to activate your smart trainer or bike-mounted power meter. Turn on the app and connect the bike/trainer to the app. Navigate to the event in the app and check in or go to the virtual start line (the process is slightly different depending on the app). Turn on the fans, grab towels, and put the remotes or other technological gear within easy reach. Get all the water and food you might need for the entire event so you don't have to get off the bike and fall behind while refilling a bottle.

6. **Save your ride.** Just as you would after a workout, be sure to save your data after the race. Whether it's a structured workout, free ride, or an e-race, the apps use the same end-of-ride steps to record and share your data, and if you forget this step, you will not be included in the race results.

like a criterium, and others are longer loops or point-to-point courses like road, gravel, and mountain bike races. They can even include virtual cobblestones and gravel, which have the effect of increasing the resistance compared to the same grade on a smooth surface. There is no standardized distance for e-racing, so you can also choose races that are similar in length to your real-world competitions or test out the intensity required for shorter events (60 minutes or shorter) and the focus and pacing necessary for long ones (2–3 hours and longer).

CHOOSE THE RIGHT CATEGORY

There is no standardized method for establishing categories for e-racing, but most competitions use either power-to-weight ratio (PWR) in watts per kilogram (W/kg) at functional threshold power (FTP) or age. Each race can set its own ranges, and most depend on the honor system for ensuring riders are competing in the appropriate categories. While choosing the right age group is simple, figuring out the right PWR category can be a bit tougher. The following is a common breakdown of e-racing categories based on PWR:

A: 4.0 or higher W/kg at FTP   **C:** 2.5 to 3.2 W/kg at FTP
B: 3.2 to 4.0 W/kg at FTP   **D:** Under 2.5 W/kg at FTP

If you are new to e-racing, err on the side of racing in a category that's too low. Because there are no entry fees for e-races, there's no financial penalty for dropping out of a race when you realize you're actually at a higher level (often known as sandbagging). Racing an easier category in the beginning can also be a good opportunity to learn how to use virtual drafting and PowerUps when you're not cross-eyed from the effort required to stay in the pack. Once you have a good understanding of how e-racing works, enter races at your true level.

KNOW THE RULES

The character and competitiveness of a race can change significantly based on the features and requirements described by the organizer. Some races allow the use of PowerUps, and others do not. Most races require a smart trainer or power meter rather than virtual power calculated from speed and the known resistance curve of a traditional/dumb trainer. Some races place restrictions on the type of bike used—not the equipment you are actually riding in your home, but the virtual equipment you are using in the app. In an effort to verify the accuracy of results and prevent cheating, some races require data from a heart rate monitor for all riders or preclude riders without heart rate data from winning.

DON'T CHEAT (INADVERTENTLY OR ON PURPOSE)

E-racing is not immune to cheating. Because the speed of your avatar in a virtual race is dependent on your stated height and weight and the accuracy of your power meter or smart trainer, riders can manipulate their data to go faster in the game.

"Weight doping" is simply increasing your PWR by saying you weigh less than you do. And in many cases, riders who record greater than 5.2 W/kg for 20 minutes or 6 W/kg for 5 minutes are flagged and removed from race results until they provide additional data to verify they are capable of that performance. Misrepresenting your height can also affect your results. Being taller increases your drag coefficient in an e-race, so over the distance of courses that feature varied terrain, saying you're 5'8" instead of 6 feet tall makes you faster at the same power output.

Some cheating is done on purpose, but a more subtle level of cheating happens inadvertently due to trainers that aren't correctly calibrated or people who entered the weight they'd like to be into their profiles instead of their actual weight. These are more errors than they are malicious, but nonetheless they can affect e-racing results.

CHOOSE THE RIGHT EQUIPMENT

In the real world, most cyclists and triathletes don't have the luxury of being able to choose between an aerodynamic bike and a lightweight bike or swap out different sets of wheels, based on the nature of a particular racecourse. In the virtual world, particularly on Zwift, the miles you ride can unlock the ability to customize your equipment. It's not just the graphics on the screen that change. The weight and aerodynamic properties of the equipment are factored into your performance on the racecourse, and in some cases can save you a minute or more in an hour of riding. Websites like Zwiftinsider.com provide updated information on the fastest frames and wheelsets for different courses.

WARM UP PROPERLY

First, gather everything you're going to need for the duration you'll be on the bike. There will be no time to hop off the bike during a Zwift race if you need water, a towel, a remote control, or a phone/keyboard for communicating. While you are warming up for a Zwift race, you can ride any other course. Before the event, you can decide to go to the start corral. Just remember that there is a front and back of the start corral based on when you get there (just like in real life).

Races in Zwift start like criteriums, cyclocross races, and short-track mountain bike races, meaning they start hard rather than with a mellow rollout like a road race. A warm-up like the example below is essential so you are ready for the hard initial effort. This example is 15 minutes as written, and I recommend starting about 20 minutes before the actual start so you have a few minutes to spin easy between the end of the warm-up and the start. This is important because to have any chance of staying in the lead group, you need to be riding at full power when the virtual flag drops. If you start pedaling when the flag drops, you'll already be far behind.

Example Warm-Up for an E-Race

---

5 minutes easy pedaling

1:30 at 65% of FTP

1:00 at 75% of FTP

0:30 at 85% of FTP

3 minutes easy pedaling

1:00 at 75% of FTP

0:30 at 100–125% of FTP

1:00 easy pedaling recovery

0:30 at 100–125% of FTP

1:00-plus of easy pedaling until the actual start. Crank up to full power in the
    30 seconds prior to the start.

START HARD

The start is one of the hardest aspects of Zwift racing. Bring your power output up as the clock ticks down to the start time so you're already at a high power when the flag drops. Be ready for a 1- to 5-minute maximum effort as riders try to split the field and create groups right away. Once the initial selections are made, the intensity comes down to a more sustainable level.

One tip for riders on smart trainers is to reduce the trainer difficulty setting before the race starts. Changing this setting—which would be more aptly named "grade accuracy"—up or down changes how much you will feel the transition from flat ground to uphill. It doesn't change the power needed to complete the climb, so it won't make you faster or slower, but lowering the trainer difficulty means a less abrupt change to the resistance as you reach a hill. This matters because racers who are not on smart trainers won't feel any difference in the resistance of their trainer based on the uphill or downhill grade in the virtual course. So, as your trainer abruptly clamps down the resistance, forcing you to adjust cadence and gearing, the riders on classic trainers continue riding smoothly. On the downhills, riders on classic trainers can (but also have to) continue riding at a high power output because the resistance on their trainer doesn't drop off. For smart trainers, the resistance drops in response to downhills, which can make it hard to generate enough power to keep from getting dropped. The solution is to reduce the trainer difficulty setting to 20–40 percent rather than the default 50 percent setting.

DRAFT WISELY

Drafting in Zwift reduces the power necessary to maintain the same speed by about 25 percent, which is similar to real life. Keep an eye on your avatar. If the speed is above 33 kilometers per hour, your avatar will "sit up" and ride on the hoods to show you are in the draft. When you are "in the drops" you are not in the draft. Note: There are some bike options that don't have a visual cue for drafting. The distance between riders matters too. Drafting benefits start at 5 meters behind the rider ahead of you and increase as you get closer. The effect of drafting is enhanced in groups larger than four riders, as you would experience in real life.

Drafting in Zwift takes some getting used to. Because there are no brakes and you can only slow down by reducing power output, you can inadvertently overtake a rider you would like to draft. You also won't feel a change in the resistance if you are using a smart trainer. Outside you can feel a drop in resistance when you're in the draft, so you know to back off the power. In Zwift, the resistance stays constant; it's just that the power necessary to maintain your position drops by 25 percent. If you don't back off, you'll surge forward out of the draft inadvertently. You also can't control when the game will move you sideways out of a draft.

Some of these drafting behaviors are sure to change as smart trainers and the game developers add features that enable virtual steering and braking.

USE POWERUPS

A whole new skill set needed for e-racing is the use of PowerUps, each of which provides a temporary benefit. As of spring 2020, there are seven PowerUps in Zwift (Table 9.1). PowerUps are awarded when you pass specific locations within a virtual route, unless you already have one you haven't used yet. The type of PowerUp you get at any location is randomly selected, and you can only have one at a time, which helps introduce some level of luck or good fortune into e-racing.

TABLE 9.1. **Zwift PowerUps**

PowerUp	Icon	Effect	Duration	Best Time to Use It
Lightweight	Feather	Reduce weight by 9.5 kg	15 seconds	On climbs
Draft Boost	Van	Increases draft effect by 50%	30 seconds	When drafting at high speeds
Aero Boost	Aero helmet	Reduces drag coefficient (CdA) by 25%	15 seconds	When riding fast with no available draft
Undraftable	Burrito	No one can draft behind you	10 seconds	When you want to attack
Cloaking	Ghost	Makes you invisible	10 seconds	When you want to attack
Large Bonus	+ 250	Unlocks experience-based features	n/a	Automatic
Small Bonus	+10			

EXPERIMENT WITH VIEWS

Zwift gives you an option of several "camera angles" ranging from your point of view, a view of your avatar from behind, and panning shots that look like you're watching yourself race on television. During a race you can use these different views to get a more complete picture for your position in the pack and what other riders are doing. Remember, unlike a real road race, you can't tell if the rider behind an avatar is about to attack or is struggling to hang on.

ANALYZE YOUR POWER FILES FROM RACES

If you are getting more involved with e-racing, it pays to dig into the power files generated from races. The performance demands for e-racing are sometimes different from what you are used to preparing for in real-world races. For instance, take a look at the duration and power output required to have a good start. If you keep getting dropped in the first 5 minutes, you can tailor your training to improve your 5-minute peak power output—something that might not be terribly important for the real-world events you compete in.

MANAGING TRAINING, FATIGUE, AND IMMUNITY

Athletes are generally healthier than sedentary people. Greater cardiorespiratory fitness reduces risk factors for heart attacks, high blood pressure, strokes, and other cardiovascular diseases. Exercise increases insulin sensitivity, reducing risk factors for developing type 2 diabetes. And the combination of exercise and eating habits helps reduce excess fat mass, which in turn reduces risk factors for obesity and obesity-related metabolic disorders, sleep apnea, and joint damage. Keep in mind, though, that improving eating habits and reducing calories matters more than increasing energy expenditure for preventing obesity.

At the same time, almost every serious athlete has personal or anecdotal experience with training hard for weeks and months only to come down with a cold right before or after an important event. We also read story after story about how elite athletes pushing the limits of human performance are walking a thin line between optimal performance and getting sick. Some take precautions like carrying their own silverware, only signing autographs with their own pen, and only drinking bottled water when traveling. The result of our personal experiences and what we observe from elite athletes is that many people believe there's a direct connection between training hard and increasing an athlete's risk of getting sick.

Training won't make you sick, at least not on its own. And while riding inside is popular year-round, the number of cyclists and triathletes riding inside increases during the winter. Similarly, the viruses that cause the flu and common cold are around all year, but winter is traditionally cold and flu season because spending more time indoors with more people increases the chance more people will come in contact with a virus. So, if you're going to be training indoors during cold and flu season, it is important to know the steps you can take to hopefully keep yourself healthy.

Knowing how to minimize your risk of infection became particularly important as we were writing the final parts of this book in early 2020, just as the COVID-19 pandemic started to take hold in the United States. While the country and the world grappled with the public health and economic consequences of protecting the population from a highly contagious respiratory virus, the relationship between exercise and immunity became a hot topic. Even as entire countries issued stay-at-home orders, closed restaurants and businesses, shut down live cultural and sporting events, and prohibited large gatherings, they encouraged people to get out and exercise because of the physical and psychological benefits of activity. At the other end of the spectrum, athletes and coaches sought clarification on the potential for high-volume and/or intensity training to suppress immune function and increase the risk for infection. The following evidence-based training recommendations for supporting immune function are not specific to COVID-19; they are meant to minimize factors that keep your immune system from operating at full capacity.

WHY ATHLETES GET SICK

The human immune system is a remarkably robust and multifaceted protection system against pathogens. When considering why athletes get sick, we have to recognize that the physical stress of training is only one component, and probably not the most important. More influential components include sleep, total energy intake, lifestyle stress, hygiene, and the number of people we come into contact with. Nevertheless, the idea that exercise suppresses the immune system comes from the observation that levels of leukocytes (white blood cells) in the bloodstream drop significantly for a period of 1–2 hours following exhaustive exercise. This led to the development of the "open window" theory, which postulated that the drop created a window for opportunistic infections.

In a 2018 research article titled "Debunking the Myth of Exercise-Induced Immune Suppression: Redefining the Impact of Exercise on Immunological Health Across the Lifespan," authors Campbell and Turner disputed the "open window" theory, asserting that the body's response to acute bouts of exhaustive exercise is to move lymphocytes to the most vulnerable places in the body, particularly the lungs. Exercise redirects immune system resources rather than suppressing or destroying them. Among other rationales, they point out that the transient drop and rapid return of circulating lymphocytes happens too quickly to be an indication that white blood cells are being produced to replace ones that have been destroyed. It is also likely that the extent of the drop isn't dramatic enough to substantially increase infection risk for an otherwise healthy individual.

If hard workouts themselves don't open up a window for opportunistic infections, we have to take a more comprehensive view of managing factors that prevent the immune system from operating at its natural best. We can divide these recommendations into three categories: training, lifestyle, and nutrition.

TRAINING RECOMMENDATIONS FOR IMMUNE SYSTEM SUPPORT

The most important training recommendation for maintaining a healthy immune system is to avoid dramatic increases in training workload. During the COVID-19 pandemic, some athletes discovered they had almost unlimited time to train due to the closure of schools and businesses. An athlete habituated to 20 hours of training per week has adapted to the physical strain on muscles, the need to take in more calories and fluids, and the need to balance the workload with recovery. Because they can handle the stress, they can maintain that workload without compromising their immune system. An athlete habituated to 8 hours of training per week shouldn't jump up to 20 hours per week just because the time becomes available. You can compensate for an isolated big week—like during a vacation or training camp—because you can rest afterward. But trying to sustain a dramatic increase is unwise because you are adding a lot of stress before you have the physiology and habits necessary to recover and adapt. To train effectively and stay healthy, follow these recommendations.

Be Conservative with Incremental Increases in Workload

For relatively inexperienced athletes (training age <5 years), weekly training workload should increase by no more than 5 percent. This includes TSS, time at intensity, and weekly overall time. More experienced athletes (with a training age of more than 5 years) may be able to increase workload by 5–10 percent per week. Because of the curvilinear nature of acquiring fitness (additional improvements get smaller and more difficult to achieve), highly fit athletes, regardless of training age, should keep incremental increases in workload under 5 percent.

Incorporate a Variety of Intensities

There isn't a particular type of cycling workout that makes you more or less susceptible to infection. High-intensity workouts won't make you sick, and long endurance rides won't protect you from an illness. It's the aggregate of your training and all the nontraining factors that will keep you healthy.

Undertake Appropriate Post-Workout Recovery Activities

Chief among these are to replenish fluids lost during training in order to maintain a positive hydration status and consume a meal rich in carbohydrate and protein within an hour after exercise.

Manage Work and Recovery Balance with Appropriate Training Dose and Density

Give your body the time it needs to recover and adapt to training stress by separating hard training sessions by sufficient rest periods. Intersperse easier training sessions with harder training sessions. And schedule more significant rest periods (2–5 days) every few weeks.

LIFESTYLE RECOMMENDATIONS FOR IMMUNE SYSTEM SUPPORT

There are 168 hours in a week, and most amateur and masters athletes train 8–20 hours per week. What you do when you're not exercising matters more than what you do immediately before, during, and after your workout.

Sleep More and Sleep Better

Sleep has a tremendous impact on immune function. According to research on the matter, healthy individuals who slept fewer than 7 hours per night were nearly three times more likely to catch the common cold than people who slept 8 hours or more. Low sleep efficiency (the amount of time in bed actually spent sleeping) further increased the risk of infection.

Reduce Stress

Acute psychological stress and acute training stress have similar effects on immune system function: they mobilize immune system resources (leukocytes or white blood cells) to increase protection against infection. Chronic stress (psychological or physiological), on the other hand, reduces the overall number of immune system cells and reduces the intensity of the "call to arms" response to pathogens. You can take the following steps to mitigate psychological stress.

Maintain daily routines, but be flexible. People thrive with structure, and disruptions to well-established routines can be very stressful. Mental health professionals recommend people create new routines rather than "go with the flow" when life and work are disrupted.

Yet, while routines and schedules are good, it is also important to be able to adapt to changing situations. Athletes typically develop a set of go-to responses to likely problems that might occur during events. Doing the same with your home and work lives is beneficial as well.

Have a support system. Everyone needs a network of people they can lean on during difficult times and celebrate with during great times. The network can include family members and friends, and it's good to include people who are not connected to your family, social group, or career. Coaches and mental health professionals can be important components of an athlete's support system.

Adopt stress-relieving behaviors. Guided meditation, mindfulness practices, yoga, and other mental and spiritual activities can help athletes disconnect from the constant noise in order to redirect negative thoughts and maintain a connection to their values and identity.

NUTRITION RECOMMENDATIONS FOR IMMUNE SYSTEM SUPPORT

The first thing that must be said is that there are no "superfoods," and it is disingenuous to promote ways to "boost" immune function through food or supplements. Nutrition is very important for supporting a robust immune system, but athletes need to be careful not to put so much faith in the power of food to protect against illness that they neglect other factors like sleep and stress. The nutrition practices that support training, general health, and immune function do not need to be complicated.

Avoid Energy Deficiency

More important than any specific food choices, consuming adequate energy to meet or slightly exceed total daily energy expenditure (basal metabolic rate + daily activities + exercise) is necessary for achieving positive training adaptations, optimizing post-workout recovery, and maintaining immune system health.

Focus on Fitness First

To perform well in endurance sports, it's advantageous to be lean and lightweight. In terms of priority, however, fitness should come first. Work to develop the best conditioning possible, which means consuming adequate energy to support your training, before turning your focus toward body weight. Most of your weight-management goals will take care of themselves when you are training with focus and feeding your body enough to have strong workouts and high-quality recovery. Creating the energy deficit necessary to proactively lose weight can hurt your training progress, hinder your recovery, and increase your risk of getting sick. That is why weight loss is best scheduled for a time when you can reduce stress elsewhere, not when you are also training hard.

Stay Hydrated

Mucous membranes in the nose and throat don't work as well when they're dry, so staying hydrated helps your natural defenses work better. Maintaining a good hydration status also facilitates normal circulation within the lymphatic system, which carries infection-fighting white blood cells throughout the body.

Eat a Varied, Whole-Food Diet Rich in Fruits, Vegetables, and Protein

No surprises here. Fresh whole foods are the best way to go. I'm happy to say that from what I've observed, the overall quality of the average endurance athlete's diet has improved over the past decade. More athletes are reducing their intakes of processed carbohydrates and are generally eating higher quality food. Whatever dietary strategy you choose, make sure you are consuming adequate total energy; that it includes plenty of carbohydrate, fat, and protein; and that it is a sustainable strategy you can stick with.

Rely on Food, Not Supplements

There are few supplements that show meaningful benefits for either preventing viral infections or easing the severity of viral infections—particularly respiratory infections. Supplementation with vitamin C, vitamin D, and probiotics is common during periods with elevated risk of viral infections, including the common cold and influenza. Whether they are effective or not in supporting immune health, large doses of antioxidants, including vitamin C, may actually diminish positive adaptations to training by reducing oxidative stress. While most supplements are generally harmless, your best bet is to consume food sources of micronutrients whenever possible, as well as sunlight for the production of vitamin D.

APPENDIX: INDOOR WORKOUTS

This appendix describes several indoor (and outdoor) cycling workouts targeting and categorized by the six abilities described in Chapter 7 and illustrated in Figure 7.2: aerobic endurance, speed skills, muscular force, muscular endurance, anaerobic endurance, and sprint power. The field tests you'll perform to establish heart rate and power zones are also included, as are combined-ability workouts. This is not intended to be a list of all of the possible workouts that can be done on an indoor cycle or trainer, but it's a good start.

In each of the ability categories that follow, only the workout's main sets are described. Workouts should always start with a warm-up and end with a cooldown. The more intense the main set of the workout, the longer the warm-up.

Workout intensities in the following workout main sets are described using the rating of perceived exertion (RPE), heart rate, and power. See Table 8.1 to establish your heart rate zones and Table 8.2 to set power zones. RPE intensity levels are illustrated in Figure 6.1. RPE is based entirely on how you feel relative to a scale of 0 (rest) to 10 (maximal effort). The power zones are based on functional threshold power (FTP), and the heart rate zones are set using functional threshold heart rate (FTHR). For an explanation of these "functional" intensity-reference points and before you do any of the following workouts, review the "Effort, Heart Rate, and Power" section in Chapter 6. Note that heart rate and power zones don't always agree—and for the most part they shouldn't, especially as fitness improves. If you have both devices, use the power meter to measure performance and the heart rate monitor to measure your effort. Both may be used along with RPE, depending on the type of workout you're doing. The power meter is the preferred intensity device for the following main sets done above zone 2. Most main sets that call for zones 1 and 2 are best done using a heart rate monitor. There are exceptions, as described below.

READING THE WORKOUT CODES

You will notice as you read through the main sets that each has a code, such as AE1, MF2, or AnE3. The first two or three letters in the code is the abbreviation of the workout's focused ability (AE = aerobic endurance, SS = speed skills, MF = muscular force, ME = muscular endurance, AnE = anaerobic endurance, and SP = sprint power). The ability tells you what the purpose of the main set is (see Chapter 7 for details). Following each ability abbreviation is a number, which reflects how difficult the main set is within its ability category. As the number increases, the main set becomes more challenging. For example, the MF2 workout is somewhat more difficult than MF1. The codes also may be used as shorthand when designing a training week, as outlined in Chapter 7. By jotting down the code of each day's workout, you save some time. And once accustomed to this system, you will know what the workout is by just glancing at the code.

FIELD TEST MAIN SET

While there is only one main set here, it produces both of the intensity reference points by which your power and heart rate training zones are set up. This is a test that should be done every 6 weeks or so to make sure your workout intensities are correct. You'll likely see little change in your heart rate zones from one test to the next, but power is likely to change considerably. These two sets of zones may overlap quite a bit when your fitness is low, but as fitness improves your power zones will rise while the heart rate zones stay about the same. The following test can be done on an indoor trainer or on the road.

T1. FTP AND FTHR TESTS

The purpose of this test is to determine your functional threshold power and functional threshold heart rate, as described in Chapter 8. Both can be determined by doing a single test. You must use a power meter to determine FTP, and you need a heart rate monitor for FTHR. Do this test following 3 to 5 days of easy training so that you come into it fresh and ready to go. This works well after a rest-and-recovery week.

This test can easily be done on an indoor cycle, traditional trainer, smart trainer, or smart bike, but realize that power in any of those cases is likely not to be the same as when on the road. Heart rate is the same regardless. Unfortunately, this means that if you have a power meter, you should do two tests—one that determines your indoor FTP and the other for your outdoor FTP. This will give you two sets of power zones, but you'll only need one set of heart rate zones.

Be aware also that using different bikes or different power meters, either indoors or on the road, is likely to result in FTPs that don't agree. The only way to be sure that your power zones are set up correctly is to use the same indoor cycle or trainer and the same power meter every time you ride.

When doing this test outdoors, find a stretch of road that is flat to slightly uphill (3 percent grade or less) with a wide bike lane, light traffic, no stop signs, and few intersections or corners. You will probably need 4 to 8 miles (7 to 15 km), depending on how fast you are and the gradient of the hill you use. Throughout the test, keep your head up so you can see ahead.

Warm up well before starting the test. Most riders need about 20 minutes. Include some high-intensity efforts near the end of the warm-up. Then recover for 3 to 5 minutes before starting the test main set. During the test, ride as if you are doing a time trial race that lasts 20 minutes. Hold back slightly in the first 5 minutes (most riders start much too fast). At the end of every 5-minute portion, decide whether to go slightly harder or easier for the next 5 minutes.

After the workout, note your average heart rate for the 20-minute test. Subtract 5 percent and you have an estimate of your FTHR. Next, use Table 8.1 to determine your heart rate training zones. To determine FTP from the same test, subtract 5 percent from your average power for the 20-minute test portion and you have an estimate of FTP. You can then use Table 8.2 to set your power training zones.

AEROBIC ENDURANCE (AE) MAIN SETS

Aerobic endurance main sets are done at the lowest intensity (zones 1 and 2, and RPE 1 to 4) of all the main sets. Their purpose is to improve your ability to use fat for fuel while developing your cardio and respiratory systems. The main benefit is improved aerobic endurance.

AE1. RECOVERY

Recovery workouts are an integral part of training throughout the season for all riders. This is the most common workout done by riders at all levels of ability. Since it is used during all warm-ups, cooldowns, recovery intervals, and on recovery rides, you should spend more time doing this main set intensity than any other.

Do this entire workout in heart rate zone 1 or in power zone 1. Heart rate is preferred. RPE for this ride is 1 to 2 (see Figure 6.1 for details on RPE). Keep it easy. The recovery ride should be of a shorter duration than your average ride. If done on the road, select a flat course. If where you live is hilly, then the indoor version of this workout is perfect and may be your only way of doing a truly easy ride. Ride primarily in the small chainring while pedaling with a comfortably high cadence.

Light exercise, such as AE1, is quite beneficial for advanced athletes who need recovery following hard workout days. But riders new to cycling may benefit more by taking the day completely off from exercise.

AE2. AEROBIC THRESHOLD

The purpose of the aerobic threshold main set is to boost aerobic fitness by improving your body's capacity for delivering and using oxygen to produce energy, largely from fat, in the muscles. It is done throughout the season but is especially important in the early Base period when developing aerobic fitness is a primary focus. As your fitness progresses, this workout is done primarily to maintain aerobic endurance.

Following a warm-up, use heart rate to gauge the intensity of this main set by keeping it mostly in low zone 2 while riding at a steady effort. RPE should be 3 to 4. Although heart rate is preferred, if you only have a power meter available, ride in low zone 2.

The aerobic threshold ride is often the longest workout in a rider's training week. As your aerobic fitness improves, it may serve as an extension of your warm-up and be preceded by another main set forming a combined-ability workout. The AE2 main set is typically 30 minutes to 2 or more hours, depending on your training goal.

This is the workout that should be used to check the progress of your aerobic fitness. After finishing this session, divide your average power by your average heart rate for the steady zone 2 portion of the ride's main set to determine your efficiency factor (EF). A gradually rising EF over the course of several weeks indicates improving aerobic endurance. It is unlikely to be a continually steady rise and will instead ratchet upward when training is progressing well. This is a perfect workout to do inside as you can do it with no interruptions due to traffic, terrain, stop signs, or weather. The resulting data can be relied on to gauge aerobic fitness progress.

SPEED SKILLS (SS) MAIN SETS

These main sets are great indoor workouts since there are no interruptions due to traffic, stop signs, or weather. The purpose of speed skills main sets is to hone your pedaling skills to improve economy. An economical rider pedals in circles with the downward force being applied very early at the top of the downstroke (around 1 o'clock), with force continuing to be applied until near the bottom of the downstroke (about 5 o'clock). On the recovery side of the stroke, the economical rider unweights the pedal. It is not pulled up—with the exception of sprinting.

In contrast, uneconomical riders pedal in squares. They apply force later in the downstroke for a very brief period by pushing straight down on the pedal from after 2 o'clock until before 4 o'clock. And then their recovery leg typically rests on the pedal on the backside of the stroke, causing the downstroke leg to have to work harder. The more economical your pedaling becomes, the less energy is wasted and therefore the more fit you become. (For more details on pedaling technique, see Chapter 2.)

Speed skills are the only main sets in which measurable intensity is not a concern, other than to keep it relatively low when doing the pedaling drills that follow. Achieving a certain intensity is not the purpose of these main sets. Use low (easy) gears when working on your skills. Straining against high resistance is counterproductive. If your legs become tired during one of the following drills, stop and take some time to recover; fatigue is the enemy of skill development, especially in the early stages of a ride.

An SS main set may accompany another main set to form a combined-ability workout. When doing this it is generally best to do the SS portion immediately following the warm-up and before the second main set. Once your skills are well developed, this main set may be done later in the workout. But again, in the early stages of skill enhancement, fatigue interferes with skill development.

SS1. SPIN-UPS

The purpose of the spin-ups workout is to improve pedaling efficiency, as indicated by the ability to comfortably maintain a high cadence. Every rider has a cadence range in which they are comfortable. By expanding that range, especially on the high-cadence end, you become more economically fit.

With your indoor cycle, traditional trainer, or smart trainer set to light resistance, and in a low (easy) gear, gradually and slowly increase your cadence for about 1 minute to your maximum spin rate. This is a cadence you can maintain without bouncing on the saddle. If you start to bounce, slow down your cadence just a little. As the cadence increases during that minute, allow your lower legs and feet to relax, especially the toes. Hold your maximum cadence for as long as possible, which will probably be only a few seconds. Recover for at least a minute. Repeat several times.

This drill is best done with a handlebar device that displays cadence. Heart rate and power measurements are not meaningful for this workout.

SS2. ISOLATED LEG

On an indoor cycle, traditional trainer, or smart trainer, using a light resistance, pedal with one leg only. The resting leg may be supported by placing the foot on a chair or stool next to the bike/trainer. Note that some indoor cycles may have a place where the nonpedaling leg may rest. If using a wheel-on trainer, be careful not to get your foot near the back wheel. In a very low (easy) gear and using only one leg, turn the cranks with a high cadence. Change legs when fatigue begins to set in. Focus on eliminating the dead spots at the top (12 o'clock) and bottom (6 o'clock) of the stroke. This workout may also be done on the road: On a flat or slightly downhill section of road, do 90 percent of the pedaling as above with one leg while the other leg "rests" but is still clipped in. Heart rate and power ratings have no significance for this workout. Remember, you will most likely not see this type of drill in a group exercise class at your local studio or gym.

SS3. 9-TO-3

As you pedal, imagine that you can drive the pedal forward from the 9 o'clock position on the back side of the stroke to 3 o'clock position on the front side without going through 12 o'clock. Obviously, you won't be able to physically do this, but that mindset will improve leg action. Use a low (easy) gear so that you can pedal with a low force at a comfortably high cadence. This will help you master the most challenging part of the pedal stroke, at the top near the 12 o'clock position.

MUSCULAR FORCE (MF) MAIN SETS

The purpose of muscular force main sets is to develop the muscular strength in your legs in order to drive the pedals down quite forcefully while staying seated. Before starting to train this ability, it is good to have become more economical in your pedaling technique so that the downstroke is long (from about 1 o'clock to 5 o'clock). The muscular force (MF) ability is especially beneficial when going uphill on the road. It also improves your power on flat terrain when trying to ride fast and steady, as in a time trial or triathlon. This is the traditional strength building that benefits all riders, indoor and outdoor—fitness, recreational, and performance riders.

Doing MF workouts is much like doing squats in the gym; the benefits are quite similar. Just as with lifting weights, you need to measure the workload to get the intensity right. The best way to gauge the intensity of these main sets is with a power meter. That power meter can be on your bicycle, on your smart trainer, or on your indoor cycle. Try to produce the highest power possible with each pedal stroke. Heart rate is not an indicator of power output. If you don't have a power meter and instead are going by perceived exertion, do the high-force portions at RPE 10—maximal effort. (One caveat: When doing these MF main sets for the first time, hold back a bit on the effort and gradually increase it as you become more experienced with this type of training. This is to reduce the likelihood of injury, especially to the knees.) The recovery after each such effort must be quite long, at least 5 minutes, since the creatine phosphate energy system being used takes about that long to restock fuel before the next high effort. A shortened recovery means that the accumulating fatigue will negatively affect the ensuing intervals, resulting in a reduced power output, which is in turn inadequate to improve muscular force. Again, think of lifting weights: If you are doing heavy 3–5 rep sets, you must take an adequate rest or you will have to reduce the working weight, which will not produce the strength gains you desire.

MF1. FLAT FORCE INTERVALS

Flat force intervals are most often done in the early Base period to prepare for the more advanced ME workouts that follow later. But they may also be done at any time during the year to build muscular strength.

Following a longish warm-up, shift to a very high gear, such as 53 × 14, and slow down so that the drive wheel nearly comes to a stop. Then, while staying seated, accelerate with as much force as you can produce to drive the pedals down. Turn the cranks for only 6 or 8 strokes so that you do a total of 3 or 4 pedal downstrokes for each leg (of course, you are alternating legs and pedaling as you normally do—it's not just pedaling with one leg). The effort should be extremely high for each downward pedal stroke. While the first couple of pedal strokes will be quite slow—around 50 rpm or lower—the cadence will gradually rise with increasing speed. But each work interval will only take a few seconds.

On an indoor cycle, traditional trainer, or smart trainer, this workout's effort in, for example, the 53 × 14 gearing would roughly equate to 2 to 3 times your FTP. How do you know what tension setting that should be on a friction or magnetic-resistance indoor cycle? Unfortunately, there is no easy answer for this; you have to experiment with your setup. If you are using your bicycle on a smart trainer, the associated app allows you to set a target wattage (as discussed in Chapter 3). Ideally, you want that wattage to be light enough that you can still turn the pedals at 50 rpm but heavy enough that you cannot last more than 6 to 7 complete revolutions as you build to 60 to 70 rpm. As you can see, this is a very narrow range that you will need in order to produce the desired physiological adaptation.

An indoor cycle would work in much the same way except that you cannot control the wattage through an app; instead, you will have to control the tension through the knob or lever. Always remember to begin on the lighter side and work your way up rather than risking an injury by starting with too much resistance.

If there is reason for concern about your knees, do only 1 set of 6 to 8 total pedal strokes and also be conservative with gear selection and effort. If at any time during this workout your knees feel unusually tender or overly stressed, stop the main set and pedal easily in a low gear for the remainder of the ride.

Warning: This is a high-risk workout. Such risky sessions can produce great fitness benefits. But doing them to the point of injury is certainly not beneficial.

Build up to doing no more than 3 sets with 6 to 8 pedal strokes in each within a workout. If you do a second or third set, recover after each by riding slowly in a low gear for at least 5 minutes before starting the next one. Do no more than 1 set the first time you do this workout. Remember, the resistance for this drill involves experimentation with gearing until you find the most appropriate setting. Err on the low-gear (easy) side at first.

Do this workout no more than twice per week, with at least 48 hours separating the sessions. As with single-leg drills, you will most likely not see this type of drill in a group ride. Flat force intervals are best done while training on your own.

MF2. HILL FORCE INTERVALS

This workout is the same as MF1, but it's done on a hill (outdoors) or a simulated hill (indoors) with the front end of your indoor cycle or bike on an indoor trainer raised. The outdoor hill will produce greater benefits due to the need to overcome gravity. Of course, gravity is not an issue indoors, but this workout will help prepare you for the posture and riding position of such workouts. As with MF1, the purpose of this main set is to develop greater neuromuscular strength. Before doing this workout on the road, you should have previously done at least 3 of the MF1 sessions and know that your knees do not complain about the high load required.

After warming up well, go to a hill if outdoors or raise the front wheel appropriately if indoors. The hill should be short (30 to 50 yards or meters) and steep (a 6 to 8 percent grade is perfect). For safety, there must be little or no traffic. You should be able to safely make a U-turn at the top and bottom of the hill.

As you coast to the base of the hill to start a set, shift to a high gear and come to a very brief, balanced stop without unclipping from the pedals. The gear you select won't be quite as high as for MF1. For example, it may be 53 × 16 instead of 53 × 14. You may have to experiment to find the right gear that allows only a cadence of around 50 rpm for the first 2 pedal strokes. Then, while staying seated, alternately drive the pedals down 3 to 4 times with each leg while otherwise pedaling in a normal manner. That's 6 to 8 total pedal strokes. Do not stand at any time on each set.

Complete up to 3 of these sets of 6 to 8 pedal strokes each in a workout. After a set, shift to a low (easy) gear and pedal gently for at least 5 minutes for recovery. Do not shorten the recovery time between sets as this will reduce the workout benefit of neuromuscular development. Be sure your legs feel recovered before doing the next set.

As with MF1, this is a high-risk, high-reward workout. At the first sign of any knee tenderness, stop the main set. Do not continue, even if the tenderness is only slight. If this happens, the next time you try it, use a lower (easier) gear.

Power, not heart rate, is the best gauge of intensity for this session, but an RPE of 10 (maximal effort) is also appropriate. Do this workout no more than twice per week, with at least 48 hours separating the sessions.

MUSCULAR ENDURANCE (ME) MAIN SETS

The purpose of the main sets in the muscular endurance ability category is to improve your sub-anaerobic threshold performance (this is also referred to as the functional threshold—see Chapter 6 for details). By improving your muscular endurance, you will become stronger and faster when around your threshold. You'll be able to ride for a longer time at a relatively high speed and power. This is especially beneficial if you participate in events such as triathlons or time trials or you just want to be able to ride faster with a higher power output.

The best way to gauge the intensity of ME main sets is with a power meter. A heart rate monitor is less effective for the shorter duration intervals that follow. For the first several minutes of an ME work interval, the heart rate will be low while rising slowly, even though the RPE that you feel may be appropriate (about 5, 6, or 7—"hard" to "really hard"). The common and inappropriate reaction of the rider using a heart rate monitor for these workouts is to greatly increase the RPE to 8 or 9 early in the work interval to force the heart rate to rise more quickly. And once the appropriate heart rate is achieved, the rider then backs off a bit. This is exactly the opposite of what should be done, though. The correct method in each of the following work intervals is to finish with a somewhat higher effort than what you started with. A power meter will help you do that better than a heart rate monitor will.

ME1. TEMPO INTERVALS

Tempo intervals is an introductory main set that should be done at least a couple of times before incorporating any of the following more challenging main sets into a training plan. At first it will be a grueling main set, but it will eventually seem easier. It's perfect for indoor rides but may also be done effectively on the road. If outside, use a mostly flat road course.

After a longish warm-up, do 3 to 5 work intervals in power zone 3 with brief recoveries in zone 1. The work intervals are fairly long, at 12 to 20 minutes, with recovery intervals that are about one-fourth as long: 3 to 5 minutes. For example, following a 16-minute work interval, recover for 4 minutes. Stay seated for each work interval.

Power is the preferred measure of intensity for this workout, but heart rate may be used since the intervals are quite long. If training only with a heart rate monitor, the work interval starts as soon as you begin pedaling hard—not when zone 3 is achieved. There will be a time lag during the interval as your heart rate is catching up. Don't try to force it to rise more quickly. When using heart rate, during the early minutes in each work interval, use an RPE of 5 to 6 (see Figure 6.1 for details on RPE) until heart rate catches up. During the recovery intervals, you should be in power zone 1 or RPE 1 to 2. If doing this main set outdoors, avoid roads with heavy traffic and frequent stop signs.

ME2. CRUISE INTERVALS

On an indoor cycle, traditional trainer, or smart trainer, or outside on a relatively flat road course, do 3 work intervals of 6 to 12 minutes' duration each. Each work interval should be done at about the anaerobic threshold: RPE 7. Power is the preferred gauge of intensity for this main set, but heart rate may be used too since the work intervals are long. For power, ride at or slightly below your FTP in zone 4. If using heart rate, gradually raise your pulse to just below your FTHR (see Table 8.1) on each work interval. With heart rate, the timed work interval portion begins as soon as the hard effort begins, not when heart rate reaches the goal intensity. As your heart rate gradually increases in the early stages of the main set, intensity is estimated based on a perceived exertion of 6 or 7 on a 10-high scale (see Figure 6.1 for details on RPE).

After each work interval, recover in zone 1 with easy pedaling for one-fourth of the duration of the preceding work interval. For example, after a 6-minute work interval, recover for 90 seconds with easy pedaling.

The first time you do this main set after a few weeks of not having done it, do a total of about 12 minutes of work intervals (for example, 2 × 6 minutes). If new to this type of main set, you should probably only do one 6-minute work interval the first time. And that should have been preceded by a few ME1 main sets in the past few weeks. Gradually, over a few such sessions, increase the total combined work interval duration to about 18 to 30 minutes (for example, 3 × 6 minutes or 3 × 10 minutes). Focus on staying relaxed during each work interval. The pedal cadence should be at a comfortable level for each work interval.

An optional variation of this main set that challenges you to work harder is to shift every 20 to 60 seconds between your normal gear and cadence for this intensity and a slightly higher (harder) gear with a somewhat lower cadence. Shift back to the previous lower gear as fatigue begins to set in at the higher gear. Another option for outdoor riding is to do the work intervals on a hill of about 3 to 5 percent grade. When doing hill cruise intervals, the recovery interval is the time it takes to turn around and descend before starting the next work interval.

ME3. SWEET SPOT INTERVALS

After a substantial warm-up, do 2 long work intervals. If on the road or a virtual route, these should be on a flat or slightly uphill (2 to 3 percent grade) course. Ride steadily, staying in the saddle for each work interval.

Each work interval should be done at 88 to 93 percent of FTP. If using a heart rate monitor, aim to plateau at about 90 to 95 percent of FTHR. The 2 work intervals are each 12, 16, or 20 minutes in duration, separated by a recovery of about one-fourth the work interval duration (for example, a 4-minute recovery between 16-minute work intervals).

ANAEROBIC ENDURANCE (ANE) MAIN SETS

The purpose of these AnE main sets is to increase your aerobic capacity (VO_2max), power, and speed and to increase the amount of time you can maintain that intensity. The main sets call for a high intensity, well above your anaerobic threshold. Don't include these in your training program until you have significantly improved your aerobic fitness by having done the preceding main sets, especially in the AE and ME ability categories, for several weeks. Use power zone 5 (see Table 8.2) for the intensity of the following workouts.

Do not use a heart rate monitor to gauge intensity for these main sets. The work intervals are so short that heart rate will rise too slowly to reflect the high intensity. If using RPE, always feel as if the work intervals are level 9 ("really, really hard").

The warm-up before an AnE workout should be long relative to the main sets described so far in this chapter, and should gradually build to a few high-intensity efforts, similar to the expected intensities of the main sets. Each of these high-intensity efforts during the warm-up is only a few seconds long, with much longer recoveries between them.

The following main sets should be done mostly while seated on your bike. Occasionally standing to shift the stress to different muscles is fine, especially if you're doing these on a hilly outdoor or virtual route. And if you're outside, be sure to find venues that have light traffic and no stop signs. Always be aware of what traffic is doing even though you are working at a high level of effort.

ANE1. VO$_2$MAX INTERVALS

After a long warm-up that finishes with several very high-intensity efforts lasting only a few seconds, do several work intervals of 30 seconds to 3 minutes each. The total high-intensity time for the work intervals should be 3 to 15 minutes. Recover after each work interval with easy pedaling in heart rate zone 1 for as long as the preceding work interval lasted. As fitness improves, gradually reduce the recovery time to half the previous work interval's duration. This progression may take several weeks. Cadence for these intervals is at the high end of your comfort range.

The first time you do this main set, start with 3 to 5 minutes of total work interval time (for example, 6 × 30 seconds) and gradually, over several sessions, build to a maximum of 15 minutes in a session (for example, 5 × 3 minutes).

A power meter is the preferred tool for measuring intensity for the work intervals. The goal intensity is power zone 5. Heart rate lag and the short work interval durations of this main set make heart rate monitors ineffective for measuring intensity. If you don't have a power meter, use an RPE of 9 ("really, really hard") on a 0–10 scale for each work interval.

Outside, these intervals may be done on a hill. The recovery intervals in this case are the duration it takes to descend the hill. Be sure to find a hill that has very light traffic and no stop signs. You should be able to make safe U-turns at the top and bottom of the hill.

ANE2. PYRAMID INTERVALS

This main set is the same as the AnE1 session, except the work intervals will increase and then decrease in duration across the session: 1-2-3-3-2-1 minutes in power zone 5. Early in the development of your anaerobic capacity, you could modify the work interval pyramids to be 1-2-2-1 minutes or 1-2-3-2-1 minutes. The recovery period after each work interval is equal to the preceding work interval duration. As your fitness improves, gradually reduce the recovery interval time to no shorter than half of the preceding work interval's duration. Cadence for these intervals is at the high end of your comfort range.

Heart rate is an ineffective gauge of intensity due to heart rate lag and the short duration of these intervals. If you don't have a power meter, use an RPE of 9 ("really, really hard") for each interval.

ANE3. GROUP RIDE

This is an unstructured ride with a group and may simulate road racing (not triathlon or time trialing). It may be done in the form of e-racing via an app and access to the internet, or it could be a B- or C-priority race in the real world. Typically, such a ride includes frequent near-maximal efforts. The goal is to push your physical and mental limits for several seconds to a few minutes many times during the ride. These powerful surges are called "matches"—highly intense anaerobic efforts—and should closely simulate the efforts of a race.

Be cautious with this workout, not only in terms of how intense it may become but also with regard to road safety if outdoors. Pay attention to traffic and other riders who may not be skilled at riding in a group. E-racing is certainly safer.

Power is the preferred metric for this main set, as heart rate is not indicative of performance.

SPRINT POWER (SP) MAIN SETS

Sprint power main sets are meant to improve your sprinting. Most of what follows are the highest intensities of all the main sets in this chapter (RPE 10) but also the shortest durations (a few seconds). Power and RPE are the only intensity metrics used here, and duration is often only the number of pedal strokes taken. These differ from the muscular force workouts that are also high intensity and short duration in that the SP main sets are done with a very high cadence and usually while standing on the pedals in simulation of a sprint.

If you are riding indoors using a wind-resistance, magnetic, or fluid trainer—or any trainer that is wobbly when standing on the pedals—*don't do these main sets*. The extremely high intensity while standing is likely to cause these types of trainers to tip over. Crashing is never good, even indoors. An indoor cycle or indoor smart bike, such as a Wattbike, can be a more stable platform for these sets.

Note that the SP1 main sets are best done before moving on to any of the other subsequent main sets, especially if you are new to cycling.

SP1. FORM SPRINTS

SP1 is the starting place for establishing the handling skills necessary to sprint effectively and efficiently. This main set is best done several times before doing the main sets that follow.

Early in the ride, after the warm-up, do 5 to 10 submaximal sprints. If on the road, use varying terrains for them: flat, uphill, and downhill. Each sprint should last 5 to 10 seconds, followed by a 3- to 5-minute recovery in zone 1. Alternate standing and sitting for the work intervals throughout this main set while focusing solely on posture and technique—*not* on power output. Since this session is done primarily for form, hold back slightly on intensity as you focus on body position relative to the bike.

Even when you are doing these indoors, the main points for sprinting posture while standing on the pedals are to (1) place your hands on the drops rather than the brake hoods, (2) bend over at the waist with the elbows slightly flexed, (3) position your butt over the nose of the saddle, (4) align your head with your hands (head is not forward of the hands), and (5) keep your head up so you can see where you are going.

Power should be in zone 5 (see Table 8.2) and RPE at 8 or 9 (see Figure 6.1). Again, note that for this main set, you are holding back just a bit on the intensity while focusing primarily on technique—especially while standing.

SP2. JUMPS

Do a thorough warm-up before this main set, as it is quite intense. The warm-up should be long relative to the warm-ups of the main sets earlier in this chapter. Near the end of the warm-up include a few sprint-type accelerations, both seated and standing, with long recoveries between them. Then, early in the main set, on a very stable trainer, indoor cycle, or indoor smart bike (or on the road), do 10 to 20 very brief surges to improve explosive power. Complete 2 to 4 sets of 5 jumps each for a total of 10 to 20 jumps in the main set. Each set involves quickly rising out of the saddle to stand on the pedals (a "jump"). And each jump is 8 to 12 revolutions of the cranks (counting both legs, so 4 to 6 strokes per leg) at a high cadence. Use good form just as you would when doing SP1. Recover by pedaling easily while seated for 1 minute following each jump and 5 minutes between sets. Power and effort should be maximal for each jump. If on the road, vary the terrain from flat to uphill to downhill, and include cornering.

SP3. GROUP SPRINTS

As with SP2, the warm-up for this main set should be relatively long and include several accelerations to maximal effort for brief periods.

Then, during a ride with a virtual group or with a partner inside (or on the road), do several 5- to 15-second race-like sprints. These are at RPE 10 while making sure good sprint form is maintained. The purpose is to simulate race intensity and tactical maneuvering. Designate sprint "finish lines," such as road signs, trees, or other landmarks. Employ all of the techniques of good form sprints (see SP1) but at a much higher intensity. Power and effort should be maximal. Recover for several minutes between sprints.

COMBINED-ABILITY MAIN SETS

While only a few combined-ability workouts are suggested here, the possibilities for such sessions are limited only by your imagination. The merging of different ability-based main sets from the six ability categories above into single workout sessions is useful for all rider types. Competitive performance riders do these mostly in the Build periods of their seasonal plans to more closely simulate the demands of racing (see Chapter 7 for more on the planning of weekly and daily training). All riders find they add variety to workouts and boost overall fitness.

The following are some commonly used combined-ability main sets. The recommended order when combining two or more of the abilities into a single workout, from the first one done in a workout to the last, is as follows:

SS → SP → MF → AnE → ME → AE

In other words, an SS main set is done first in a workout (after warming up) and an AE done last (before cooling down). So a sprint power (SP) main set should usually precede an anaerobic endurance (AnE) main set when they are combined into one session. (I say "usually" because there are always exceptions, as you will see below, but they are rare.) This order has to do with the accumulated effect of fatigue on performance during a ride. Fatigue's effects on performance in subsequent main sets can be significant. Yet there may be times when you want to do a workout main set when fatigued because that is to be expected during race-like events. However, note that speed skills always come first in a combined workout because fatigue significantly conflicts with skill development. By doing the SS portion first, your body can execute the technique better and your skills are more likely to improve. And also note that an aerobic endurance set comes last when combining abilities as building this ability is less affected by fatigue than are the other abilities. In fact, an underlying purpose of AE is to reduce the effect of fatigue on performance by becoming better at coping with it (see "Efficiency Factor" in Chapter 8).

With all of this in mind, the following are but a few examples of combined-ability main sets.

SS1 + AE2

After the warm-up, follow the guidelines for the SS1 main set to refine pedaling skills; you'll do several minutes of spin-ups in a very low (easy) gear. Gradually increase to a very high cadence on each brief spin-up while focusing on total body relaxation. Each spin-up should last only a few seconds. When you find you can no longer relax or your pedal stroke becomes sloppy, it's time to stop the spin-ups and move on to the AE2 portion of the ride. For this main set, ride steadily in heart rate zone 2, as described in the AE2 instructions, for the remainder of the workout. This will help boost your aerobic endurance. To see how your aerobic fitness is coming along, when the workout is done, divide your average power by your average heart rate for the steady AE2 zone 2 portion of the ride to determine your efficiency factor. Over several weeks you should see it increase, which tells you that your aerobic endurance is improving. Another option for this workout is to alternate spin-ups and steady zone 2 riding. Within a steady AE2 main set, insert a single spin-up every few minutes. When doing these, concentrate on relaxation and a smooth, circular pedal stroke.

MF1 + AE2

Following a long and progressively harder warm-up, do 1 to 3 sets with 6 to 8 maximal-effort pedal strokes in each set, as described above in main set MF1. Stay seated for each. The purpose is to build muscular strength so you apply a greater force to the pedal. These should be all-out efforts at an RPE of 10. Recover for 5 minutes after each maximal effort by pedaling easily in heart rate zone 1. (If you feel any tenderness in your knees, stop the MF1 main set and go on to the AE2 portion of the workout.) After the last 5-minute recovery, ride in zone 2 for the remainder of the main set before doing a brief cooldown. After the ride, determine your efficiency factor: Divide your average power for the AE2 main set by your heart rate for the same portion.

ME1 + AE2

Warm up well and then do 1 to 3 work intervals of 6 minutes' duration each in power zone 3 (RPE 5 to 6) with 90-second recovery intervals between them. Recover in heart rate zone 1 (RPE 1 or 2) for about 5 minutes after the last work interval before beginning a steady AE2 main set; ride in heart rate zone 2. After the ride, determine your efficiency factor: Divide your average power for the AE2 main set by your average heart rate for the main set. Your EF should increase over several weeks, indicating that your aerobic endurance fitness is improving.

SP2 + ANE1

Following a long warm-up including a few very brief, maximal efforts near the end, do 2 to 4 sets of 5 jumps each, as described above in main set SP2. Focus on good technique for each sprint (see main set SP1 for a description of sprint technique). Then, after a 5-minute or so easy recovery spin in heart rate zone 1, do a total of 5 to 15 minutes of work intervals, with each lasting 30 seconds to 3 minutes in power zone 5 or RPE 9. The recovery intervals after each should be of an equal duration or somewhat shorter, as described in main set AnE1. You may also substitute main set AnE2 for the AnE1 portion of this workout. Finish the workout with a long, very easy cooldown in heart rate zone 1.

ANE1 + ME2

This is a challenging workout and should only be attempted by a highly experienced rider. Be sure to warm up well before starting the high-intensity portions that follow. The warm-up should be relatively long and include several brief high-intensity efforts. Next, do the AnE1 main set. It's generally best not to do as many of these AnE1 intervals as when done as a stand-alone main set as the combination of these two abilities is quite stressful. Recover for 5 to 10 minutes in zone 1 following the AnE intervals before starting the ME2 portion. For this second main set, do 1 to 3 work intervals of 6 to 12 minutes' duration each with recovery intervals that are one-fourth the duration of the preceding work interval. You may also substitute main set ME1 for the last high-intensity portion of this workout. Another option for this workout is to alternate short (30 seconds to 3 minutes) AnE1 work intervals with long (6 to 12 minutes) ME2 work intervals. With this option, the recovery interval after each work interval is the duration of the previous work interval. For example, following a 30-second AnE1 work interval, recover for 30 seconds before doing a 6-minute ME2 work interval. This alternating main set option makes for a very challenging workout. You should have completed a few stand-alone AnE and ME sessions in the previous weeks before attempting this workout.

SS1 + ME1 + AE2

An option for the more experienced rider is to do a workout consisting of parts of three or even four main sets in a single workout. Here is but one example.

After the warm-up, work on sprint skills by doing main set SS1. Focus only on sprint technique (see SS1 for the details of sprint technique). Immediately following that main set do ME1 intervals in power zone 3 or RPE 5 to 6; see the interval details in the ME1 description. Recover in heart rate zone 1 for 5 minutes or so and then begin the AE2 main set. The first time you do such a three-part ride, it's wise to reduce the number of ME1 work intervals from what you may do in the same main sets done as stand-alone workouts.

SP1 + ANE1 + ME2 + ANE1 + SP3

This is a very challenging five-part workout intended to be only done by highly advanced riders. Note the exception to the rule here about having SP main sets precede ME and AnE main sets, which are also in the reverse order from what was suggested earlier. The reasoning here is that in a cycling road race or criterium, the last four main sets often occur in this order. While arranging the main sets this way may not be best for developing each ability, this race-like format is effective for preparing the rider for competition, especially after all of the individual abilities have been well established in the earlier part of the season.

Be sure to warm up well. As a part of the latter stages of the warm-up, work on sprint technique by following the instructions for SP1 main sets. Then go immediately into AnE1 main set intervals. The first time you do this workout, keep the total high-intensity time for work intervals at a very low number, such as 5 to 10 minutes. Immediately following the AnE1 intervals, begin ME2 intervals. Again, hold down the total work interval duration the first time you do this session. Then return to AnE1 work intervals again before finishing with a few SP3 group sprints (or SP2 if no group is available).

ACKNOWLEDGMENTS

Joe Friel

This book would not have been possible without the assistance of many others.

First, I would like to thank Jim Rutberg for his in-depth contributions to this project and his carefully considered thoughts on the book's organization and on much of the writing. His knowledge and personal experience with the technology and equipment necessary for riding inside was extremely valuable. I owe you big time, Jim!

I am also especially grateful for the guidance of Andy Read, the acquisitions editor for the publisher, VeloPress. Andy took on the project as soon as I proposed it, nurtured the concept, and helped guide the details of the manuscript for over a year with many iterations. His questions and suggestions helped to focus me and take this book from an idea to a finished project. Thanks, Andy!

Working closely with Andy were several editors who made my rough concepts and descriptions readable. That includes Sarah Gorecki, Vicki Hopewell, and Kara Mannix of VeloPress along with copyeditor Gretel Hakanson and proofreader Kelly Anne Lenkevich. Thank you all!

My good friend Tim Cusick of WKO software was especially helpful in his assistance in explaining the differences between power production on a bike ridden inside and out. As always, thanks for your insights, Tim!

I also want to thank the many cyclists and triathletes who have given me personal feedback on my inside workouts that are featured in the appendix of this book. Thanks!

Jim Rutberg

Throughout my career, I have been fortunate to work with and learn from great coaches and hopefully to make sports science and endurance training more accessible to athletes at all levels. Virtually every athlete, coach, and outdoor sports author I know has Joe Friel's books on his or her shelf, and I'm honored to contribute to one. Thank you to Joe and to Andy Read, acquisitions editor at VeloPress, for their confidence and support, and for asking me to be a part of the project. And thank you to Leslie, Oliver, and Elliot for putting up with me during the process.

REFERENCES

Chapter 4: Setting Up Your Space

Bongers, Coen C. W. G., Maria T. E. Hopman, and Thijs M. H. Eijsvogels. "Cooling Interventions for Athletes: An Overview of Effectiveness, Physiological Mechanisms, and Practical Considerations." *Temperature: Medical Physiology and Beyond* 4, no. 1 (2017): 60–78. https://doi.org/10.1080/23328940.2016.1277003.

Cheung, Stephen S. "Interconnections Between Thermal Perception and Exercise Capacity in the Heat." *Scandinavian Journal of Medicine and Science in Sports* 20, no. S3 (2010). https://doi.org/10.1111/j.1600-0838.2010.01209.x.

Jeffries, O., and M. Waldron. "The Effects of Menthol on Exercise Performance and Thermal Sensation: A Meta-Analysis." *Journal of Science and Medicine in Sport* 22, no. 6 (2019): 707–715. https://www.doi.org/10.1016/j.jsams.2018.12.002.

Peiffer, Jeremiah J., and Chris R. Abbiss. "Influence of Environmental Temperature on 40 km of Cycling Time-Trial Performance." *International Journal of Sports Physiology and Performance* 6 (2011): 208–220. https://doi.org/10.1123/ijspp.6.2.208.

Chapter 5: Four Ways to Ride Inside

Irwin, B. C., J. Scorniaenchi, N. L. Kerr, J. C. Eisenmann, and D. L. Feltz. "Aerobic Exercise Is Promoted When Individual Performance Affects the Group: A Test of the Kohler Motivation Gain Effect." (2012). https://www.doi.org/doi:10.1007/s12160-012-9367-4. Retrieved from http://krex.ksu.edu.

Chapter 9: Putting It All Together

Campbell, John P., and James E. Turner. "Debunking the Myth of Exercise-Induced Immune Suppression: Redefining the Impact of Exercise on Immunological Health Across the Lifespan." *Frontiers in Immunology* 9 (2018). https://doi.org/10.3389/fimmu.2018.00648.

Centers for Disease Control and Prevention. "Coronavirus Disease 2019 (COVID-19)." http://www.cdc.gov/coronavirus/2019-nCoV/index.html.

Cohen, Sheldon, William J. Doyle, Cuneyt M. Alper, Denise Janicki-Deverts, and Ronald B. Turner. "Sleep Habits and Susceptibility to the Common Cold." *Archives of Internal Medicine* 169, no. 1 (2009): 62. https://doi.org/10.1001/archinternmed.2008.505.

Gleeson, Michael. "Immune Function in Sport and Exercise." *Journal of Applied Physiology* 103, no. 2 (2007): 693–699. https://doi.org/10.1152/japplphysiol.00008.2007.

Simpson, Richard, John P. Campbell, Maree Gleeson, Karsten Krüger, David C. Nieman, David B. Pyne, James E. Turner, and Neil P. Walsh. "Can Exercise Affect Immune Function to Increase Susceptibility to Infection?" *Exercise Immunology Review* 26 (2020): 8–22.

Walsh, Neil P. "Recommendations to Maintain Immune Health in Athletes." *European Journal of Sport Science* 18, no. 6 (2018): 820–831. https://www.doi.org/10.1080/17461391.2018.1449895.

Walsh, Neil P. "Nutrition and Athlete Immune Health: New Perspectives on an Old Paradigm." *Sports Medicine* 49, no. S2 (2019): 153–168. https://www.doi.org/10.1007/s40279-019-01160-3.

Walsh, Neil P., Michael Gleeson, David B. Pyne, David C. Nieman, Firdaus S. Dhabhar, Roy J. Shephard, Samuel J. Oliver, Stéphane Bermon, and Alma Kajeniene. "Position Statement Part Two: Maintaining Immune Health." Loughborough University (2011). Journal contribution. https://hdl.handle.net/2134/10586.

Walsh, Neil P., Michael Gleeson, Roy J. Shephard, Maree Gleeson, Jeffery A. Woods, Nicolette Bishop, Monika Fleshner, Charlotte Green, Bente K. Pedersen, Laurie Hoffman-Goete, Connie J. Rogers, Hinnak Northoff, Asghar Abbasi, and Perikles Simon. "Position Statement Part One: Immune Function and Exercise." Loughborough University (2011). Journal contribution. https://hdl.handle.net/2134/10584.

ABOUT THE AUTHORS

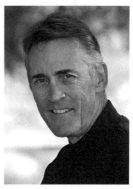

Joe Friel is a lifelong athlete and holds a master's degree in exercise science. He has trained and conferred with amateur and professional endurance athletes from a wide variety of sports since 1980. His coaching experience and research led him to cofound TrainingPeaks .com in 1999 with son Dirk Friel and friend Gear Fisher.

Friel is semiretired from one-on-one coaching and now updates emerging top-level coaches from several sports on best practices for preparing endurance athletes for competition, work that regularly takes him to coaching seminars around the world. He also consults with corporations in the sports and fitness industry and with national Olympic governing bodies worldwide. His *Training Bible* books for road cyclists and triathletes are used by several national sports federations to train their coaches.

Friel's philosophy and methodology for training athletes was developed over more than 40 years and is based on his strong interest in sports science research and his experience training hundreds of athletes with a wide range of abilities. His views on matters related to training for endurance sports are widely sought and have been featured in such publications as *VeloNews*, *Bicycling*, *Outside*, *Runner's World*, *Women's Sports & Fitness*, *Men's Fitness*, *Men's Health*, *American Health*, *Masters Sports*, the *New York Times*, *Triathlete*, and more.

To connect with Joe and find more information on training, go to his blog at joefrielsblog.com and follow him on Twitter at @jfriel.

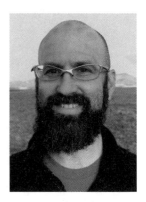

Jim Rutberg is the owner of Rutberg Communications and has been an athlete, coach, and content creator focusing on outdoor sports, endurance coaching, and cycling events for more than 20 years. He is the media director and a coach for CTS, and coauthor, with Chris Carmichael, of *The Ultimate Ride, Chris Carmichael's Food for Fitness, Chris Carmichael's Fitness Cookbook, The Carmichael Training Systems Cyclist's Training Diary, 5 Essentials for a Winning Life, The Time-Crunched Cyclist,* and *The Time-Crunched Triathlete.* He also coauthored *Training Essentials for Ultrarunning* with Jason Koop and has written innumerable web and magazine articles. His work has appeared in *Bicycling, Outside, Men's Health, Men's Journal, VeloNews, Inside Triathlon,* and more. A graduate of Wake Forest University with a bachelor's degree in exercise science and former elite-level cyclist, Jim resides in Colorado Springs, Colorado, with Leslie, and their two sons, Oliver and Elliot.

VISIT
VELOPRESS.COM

for more on running, cycling, triathlon,
swimming, ultrarunning,
yoga, recovery, mental training,
health and fitness, nutrition, and diet.

SAVE $10
ON YOUR FIRST ORDER

Shop with us and use coupon code
VPFIRST during checkout.

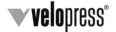

ALSO AVAILABLE FROM VELOPRESS

FIND NEW SPEED

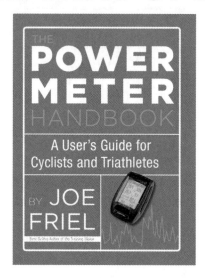

In *The Power Meter Handbook*, Joe Friel offers cyclists and triathletes a simple user's guide to using a power meter for big performance gains. In simple language, the most trusted coach in endurance sports makes understanding a power meter easy, no advanced degrees or tech savvy required. Cyclists and triathletes will master the basics to reveal how powerful they are. Focusing on their most important data, they'll discover hidden power, refine their pacing, and find out how many matches they can burn on any given day. Once they understand the fundamentals, Friel will show how to apply his proven training approach to gain big performance in road races, time trials, triathlons, and century rides.

The Power Meter Handbook: A User's Guide for Cyclists and Triathletes by Joe Friel

Paperback with charts and tables throughout
6" × 8", 192 pp., $16.95, 978-1-934030-95-0

Available in bookstores, cycling, tri, and running shops, and online.

Learn more about VeloPress books at
velopress.com/books/the-power-meter-handbook/